THE PEOPLE
WHO MADE THE
PILL

THE PEOPLE WHO MADE THE

PILL

AN IN-DEPTH LOOK AT THE CHARACTERS BEHIND ORAL CONTRACEPTION

DR. DAVID M. C. HISLOP

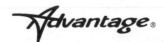

Published by Advantage, Charleston, South Carolina.
Member of Advantage Media Group.

ADVANTAGE is a registered trademark and the Advantage colophon is a trademark of Advantage Media Group, Inc.

Printed in the United States of America.

ISBN: 978-159932-287-2
LCCN: 2011942690

This publication is designed to provide accurate and authoritative information in regard to the subject matter covered. It is sold with the understanding that the publisher is not engaged in rendering legal, accounting, or other professional services. If legal advice or other expert assistance is required, the services of a competent professional person should be sought.

Advantage Media Group is proud to be a part of the Tree Neutral® program. Tree Neutral offsets the number of trees consumed in the production and printing of this book by taking proactive steps such as planting trees in direct proportion to the number of trees used to print books. To learn more about Tree Neutral, please visit **www.treeneutral.com**. To learn more about Advantage's commitment to being a responsible steward of the environment, please visit **www.advantagefamily.com/green**

Advantage Media Group is a leading publisher of business, motivation, and self-help authors. Do you have a manuscript or book idea that you would like to have considered for publication? Please visit **www.amgbook.com** or call **1.866.775.1696**

Acknowledgments

T he author wishes to extend his sincerest thanks to Adam Witty, Chief Executive Officer of Advantage Media Group, and to the editorial staff of Advantage for their energy and enthusiasm in producing this work. Specifically, he wishes to thank Brooke White for her work in editing, and graphic designer, George Stevens, for his attention to graphs and other illustrations.

Special thanks are due to Melba Moss, former chief librarian at Port Huron Hospital, and now branch librarian of the St. Clair County Library, and to David Smith, reference librarian at St. Clair County Library, each for their work in securing copies of scientific papers, so essential to the scope of this work.

In addition, I would like to express my gratitude to Professor Emeritus, Roy A. Olofson, of the Department of Chemistry at Pennsylvania State University, for his kindness in introducing me to the university library collection of data on Russell Marker.

Table of Contents

Introduction

Too few of us is given the opportunity to change the course of human thought and action. Such requires not only foresight as to the direction of change, but the conviction that the direction is appropriate. To effect change requires tenacity, courage and willpower, aided by intellectual capacity. This is the story of the development of the oral contraceptive pill, an invention that has quietly revolutionized our attitudes to sexual behavior. Of even greater importance, it has empowered our ability to control reproduction in an effective and reversible manner. It has provided women with undreamed-of career opportunities by freeing them from unwanted and untimely pregnancy. The advent of the oral contraceptive has caused society to change attitudes toward the whole field of reproduction. For, after all, if reproduction may be controlled temporarily, why not in permanent fashion? Thus society has come to accept male and female sterilization. If society has less readily accepted abortion, the latter has at least been made legal.

The individuals who drove the development of the oral contraceptive to its successful conclusion include a collection of characters who, were they fictitious, would stretch credibility. From the single-mindedness of reformer Margaret Sanger to the non-conformist behavior of Russell Marker to the apostasy of devout Catholic John Rock, each was an outlier in the norms of human behavior. Each had, in varying amounts, the aforementioned virtues of tenacity and courage. All were endowed with intellectual capacity far above the average. It is to these individuals that this book is dedicated.

While the first chapter is devoted to Anthony Comstock, this anomaly must be excused by the reader. He was not among the group who furthered the development of the oral contraceptive pill. Quite the contrary. His powerful position as the special agent of the post-master general provided him with a monopoly on the legal determination of obscenity and gave him the role of final arbiter. As such, he and the Comstock laws, of which he was the progenitor, presented an almost insuperable barrier to the agents for change. His biography, however, is essential for the reader's understanding of the social and legal environment in which they worked.

It is not the purpose of this book to follow the convoluted currents of the political, religious and social tides of change during the 100 years or so of the birth control movement, but only as they were relevant to the careers of our characters. Such history has been dealt with in much detail by professional historians. For example, we have not pursued the career of Margaret Sanger after the 1936 watershed decision of *One Package...of Rubber Pessaries*, which over-turned at least the federal proscriptions of birth control, for thereafter, while consolidating the political advantages of the decision, the history of the pill is removed from her direct jurisdiction until the brief episode of her financial support of Pincus' research in the early 1950s.

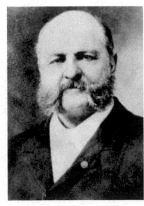

CHAPTER ONE

The Reformer
Anthony Comstock

"To promote a woman to bear rule, superiority, dominion, or empire above any realm, nation, or city is repugnant to Nature, contumely to God, a thing most contrarious to His revealed will and approved ordinance; and finally it is the subversion of good order, of all equity and justice.... Woman in her greatest perfection was made to serve and obey man, not to rule and command him."[1]

John Knox, 1558

On March 3, 1873, Congress passed a bill targeting obscenity, pornography, abortion and contraception that was quickly signed into law by then-President Grant. The progenitor and virulent prosecutor of this law was the young Anthony Comstock, only four days shy of his 29th birthday. So

---

1   John Knox was a prominent Scottish Protestant reformer. It was his misfortune to live at a time when the heads of European states were women viz. Mary, Queen of Scots, Elizabeth of England, and Catherine de Medici, Queen Regent of France, while Spain, until recently, had been governed by Ferdinand and Isabella as joint rulers. It did not help Knox that all but Elizabeth were Catholic.

strong was his association with this legislation that it became known as the Comstock Act.

Who was Anthony Comstock? Born on a rural farm in New Canaan, Connecticut, on March 7, 1844, he was one of 10 children borne by Polly Lockwood Comstock, of whom seven survived into adulthood.

His father, Thomas, a man of substance, owned 160 acres of farmland as well as two sawmills. Both parents were of Puritan stock. Anthony was deeply attached to his mother, whose memory he honored throughout his life, notwithstanding that Polly died when he was a mere 10 years of age. For all of his life, Comstock was deeply religious, as evidenced not only by his behavior but also by his sporadically written diary, where he confided his trials of pervasive temptation always preempted by his faith in God and Jesus. Reading between the lines, it seems Anthony had guilt feelings over his adolescent sexual fantasies and self-stimulation. But his was a religion of sanctimony unleavened by amity or compassion. He envisaged the devil as an anthropomorphic entity with whom he was engaged in a lifelong struggle. Apart from a minor teenage infraction, he abstained from alcohol, and was a strict observer of the Sabbath, hesitant even to engage in any of his many travels on a Sunday.

He was a man of unquestionable physical courage. Trumbull, in his biography, describes how, as an 18-year-old, Comstock alone faced off against a rabid mastiff hound of great size that had terrorized the village, fatally wounding it with a single shot. Acting alone he later surreptitiously gained access to a local gin mill that had a reputation for selling liquor to women and children, and which the local sheriff feared to close despite the absence of a liquor license. After surveying the building, Comstock returned a few nights later, broke in, and emptied on the floor all of its liquor receptacles. With seemingly little fear of reprisal, he left a notice threatening to have the building torn down should the owners attempt renewal of their business. It is recorded that the owners, a consortium of New Yorkers, quietly left the scene.

He enlisted in the Union Army at the age of 17 to replace his older brother Samuel, who had died heroically at Gettysburg. In the military, he was distressed to find that he was required to work on Sundays and that swearing, chewing of tobacco, and drinking were common. Whisky was issued to the men at sporadic intervals, but Anthony would pour his into the ground rather than donate it to his fellows. Although such actions could scarcely have endeared him to his comrades in arms, he was by all accounts an exemplary soldier. It is recorded that he was promoted to corporal within a week of enlistment. In his diary entry of March 20, he notes that a military inspector took his rifle to the tent of the major, where it was shown as the best-cleaned rifle of his company.

Comstock had little sense of the aesthetic. He rarely attended theater other than to seek condemnation of its products. Although he records in his Army diary how he was smitten with a sense of beauty by the sight of the moon on water, an experience of nearly ubiquitous appeal, he almost instantly writes that the experience bordered on sin, that the devil might be lurking behind the moon, and that the silver sheen might have emanated from the pits of hell.

Physically, Anthony Comstock was an imposing figure. His sympathetic biographer Trumbull reports that he was 5' 10" tall and weighed 220 pounds. He was deep-chested, broad-shouldered and bull-necked, with legs that were likened to tree trunks. These physical assets were useful in his not-infrequent physical encounters with alleged malefactors. However, on one occasion, at the age of 30, when attempting to arrest a dealer in erotic books, Comstock was left scarred for life when the dealer, Conroy by name, thrust a dirk into his face.

His private life was unassailable. Following his discharge from the Army and after some months, he went to work in New York at the dry goods store of Cochran, McLean, where he saved enough money to afford marriage. In January 1871, he entered into wedlock with Margaret Hamilton, a wraith of a woman weighing 80 pounds and some 10 years his senior. She was the daughter of an elder of the Presbyterian Church. But the marriage was felicitous. One reads of Comstock's return one afternoon to his empty home to find an unfinished dress, which he promptly completes before the return of his wife. One cannot read without compassion of the death of their only child, daughter Lillie, in June of 1972, at the age of six months; of his adoption of Adele, a waif whose mother died in childbirth and to whom he remained loyal despite her mental retardation and troubling personality; of his provision of care in his home for Jennie, the chronically bedridden sister of his wife. Financially he was incorruptible. In the early '80s he mounted a campaign against the Louisiana Lottery, a hugely profitable enterprise sustained by the bribery of officials and police agencies, not to mention the press, where adverts for the lottery were a major source of income. It was reputed to net $5,000 per day. A representative of this enterprise first offered to support Comstock's recently formed Committee for the Suppression of Vice to the tune of $25,000 in exchange for his goodwill. Incredulous of Comstock's refusal, he next offered a salary of $20,000 per year to subsidize a five-year sojourn in Europe, where he and his wife could "broaden their outlooks." This, too, was rejected. Ultimately, Comstock forced the closure of this and other lotteries by a stringent federal law passed in 1893.

Laws restricting obscenity were not new to the United States. Most were based on English common law, which had long been in effect. In New York State, the board members of the YMCA had finally been successful in 1868 in securing the state legislature's passage of an anti-obscenity bill. In 1882, Comstock imprisoned four individuals found guilty under its terms. Comstock was able to enlist the help and enthusiasm of the board of the New York YMCA, several of whose members were wealthy. For example, Samuel Colgate, of toothpaste fame, was at one time a chairman. The board was persuaded to form the Committee for the Suppression of Vice, modeled after a similar agency in Great Britain.

In the fall of 1872, in what became a sensational case, Comstock brought charges of obscenity against the twin sisters Victoria Woodhull and Tennessee Claflin, which excited a great deal of attention. The sisters were publishers of a newspaper called the Woodhull and Claflin's Weekly, which had achieved some notoriety for its advocacy not only of women's rights and suffrage, but also free love. (Woodhull, in fact, later became the first woman to run for the presidency of the United States under the auspices of the Equal Rights Party). The public furor arose over an item issued in the newspaper of 2nd November, 1872, alleging the adultery of a famous and well-respected minister of the church, the Rev. Henry Ward Beecher. Whether the allegations were true or not, and the preponderance of evidence suggests that they were, Comstock took the tack that the mere publication of such material constituted obscenity. At first he proffered charges in the state courts, but these were dismissed by the presiding judge, whom Comstock accused of venality. On the same day, he brought charges under the federal statute of 8th June, 1872, which contained a provision entailing the mailing of obscene material, and had the sisters arrested. The Claflin sisters, both young and attractive, were jailed in Manhattan's Ludlow Street prison, refusing bail for four weeks until released in December. So sensational was the November 1872 issue of the Weekly that, although suppressed, clandestine copies were later sold privately at a premium. In January, when this came to the attention of Comstock, he ordered copies of the publication to be sent to him via the post office using a false name and address. Upon receipt, he once more had the sisters arrested and jailed accusing them of mailing obscene materials. Included in the arrests was Col. James Blood, the husband of Victoria. Once more they were released and once more, at the insistence of Comstock, they were arrested in February of '83.

When in June they came to trial, the case was shortly dismissed. Although the law proscribed the mailing of obscene materials it did not specifically include newspapers, which provided a loophole for the sisters, a loophole that Comstock was shortly to close.

Absurd as the entire issue might seem to modern eyes, it gives evidence of Comstock's sedulous tenacity and zealotry. The huge publicity drew attention to his cause, moving him from obscurity into the public eye, but caused the YMCA board to distance themselves from his actions, preferring him to pursue his work through the Committee for Suppression of Vice; this provided them with anonymity.

In the early year of 1872, Comstock had been busy on the political scene. He deemed the New York statute of 1872, although harsh by modern standards, to be insufficiently strong for his purposes. Through the earnest endeavors of the Committee for the

Suppression of Vice, a new bill for federal consideration had been carefully prepared with the best legal advice. Despite the committee's reservations about the Weekly, the Woodhull and Claflin controversy, and press criticism, Comstock persuaded it to promote the bill and energetically pursued its passage. The timing was not propitious. Congress was turbulently involved in a scandal over allegations of corruption in the Crédit Mobilier financing of the Union Pacific Railroad. For all the turmoil, it is a paradox that Comstock was insouciant of the overt venality associated with the issue, only agonizing over the delay in the passage of his own proposed legislation. Toward this end, he importuned congressional representatives, displaying, to their horror, his multiple, lurid and vile examples of contemporary pornography.

The proposed bill, in addition to outlawing obscenity, without defining it, outlawed contraception and rendered it unlawful to provide written information on the subject. Besides lacking any definition of obscenity, the bill also rendered it illegal to mail so-called obscene literature, articles and other items. In mid-February, Comstock appeared before the Committee on Post Offices and Post Roads, where the members unanimously consented to his bill. After many vicissitudes, the bill was passed early on the morning of 3rd March 1873, and President Grant signed it into law the same day.

Comstock was elated. His victory was enhanced when, on 6th March, he was given a commission as Special Agent from the postmaster general. In effect, this commission made him the sole arbiter of what constituted pornography in United States postal shipments, an immense monopoly of power that he subsequently abused in the furtherance of his views. Here are the more significant sections of the law as it was published:

"Be it enacted…that whoever, within the District of Columbia or any of the Territories of the United States…shall sell, or to lend, or to give away, or in any manner exhibit, or shall otherwise publish or offer to publish in any manner, or shall have in his possession, for any such purpose or purposes, an obscene book, pamphlet, paper, writing or advertisement, circular, print, drawing or other representation, figure or image on or of paper or other material, or any cast instrument, or other article of an immoral nature, or any drug or medicine, or **any article whatever, for the prevention of conception, or for causing unlawful abortion** or shall advertise the same for sale, or shall write or print, or cause to be written or printed any card, circular book, pamphlet, advertisement or notice of any kind, stating when, where, how or of whom or by what means any of the articles in this section…can be purchased or obtained or shall manufacture, draw, or print, or in any wise make any of such articles, shall be deemed guilty of a misdemeanor, and on conviction thereof in any court of the United States…he shall be imprisoned at hard labor in the penitentiary for not less than six months nor more than five years for each offense, or fined not less than one hundred dollars nor more than two thousand dollars with costs of court."

The Post Office laws were amended so that under Section 148, articles 14 and 16 would then read as follows:

"14) Any person who shall knowingly deposit or cause to be deposited for mailing or delivery any of the hereinbefore-mentioned articles or things, or any notice, or paper containing any advertisement relating to the aforesaid article or things…

16) shall be deemed guilty of a misdemeanor and, on conviction thereof, shall, for every offense be fined not less than

one hundred dollars nor more than five thousand dollars, or imprisoned at hard labor not less than one year nor more than ten years or both at the discretion of the judge."

As noted, it does not contain any definition of obscenity, so that Comstock became virtually the sole judge and determinant. The law included a paragraph making it illegal to possess any article for the prevention of conception or for causing abortion or of advertising such items for sale. No such article could be mailed through the United States Post Office. The penalties, besides substantial fines, could amount to as much as ten years of hard labor.

Comstock was now cut loose on society, armed with a restrictive law and his own prejudices. One of his most famous cases involved a certain Madame Restell (Ann Trow Lohman b.1812-d.1st April, 1878). Mme Restell was the widow of "Dr." Charles Lohman. She had acquired notoriety as an abortionist and peddler of contraceptive medications, which she advertised in the press, providing mail orders. It is also probable that she performed midwifery services. Certainly she advertised herself as "Madame Restell, female physician and professor of midwifery." Whatever her precise vocational forays, they were certainly lucrative. When her step-daughter Caroline was married in 1854, it is said that she received $50,000 for her European honeymoon. In 1864, Restell moved into an expensive home on 5th Avenue. At her demise, she left an estate that exceeded $1 million, not to mention a $3,000-per-month annuity for Caroline.

Even before she came to the attention of Comstock, Restell had experienced several legal difficulties. In 1841, she was tried and convicted of causing a death from abortion. In 1846, she was put up for trial after being accused of having forcibly adopted out the infant of a young patient against the woman's will. She was acquitted, and there was suspicion that she had bribed various officials to secure her release. In 1847, she was again accused and arrested for performing an unlawful abortion. The trial drew huge attention in the press, but Restell was found guilty on a lesser charge. She spent a year in New York's notorious Blackwell Prison, where descriptions of the leniency of her treatment caused a public scandal.

In the spring of 1878, Comstock, lying unscrupulously, presented himself to Restell as a customer in search of contraceptive materials for a wife "in trouble." Appealing more to Restell's compassion rather than her concupiscence, he made his purchases. He followed this by securing a search warrant. Having found sufficient evidence at her home, despite the maneuverings of her attorney, he had Restell arrested. She failed in her attempt to buy off Comstock with a bribe of $40,000, an immense sum in those days. She was scheduled for trial on 1st April for "possession of articles used for immoral purposes." On the morning of the trial, at the age of 67 years, Ann Lohman (Restell) slit her throat with a carving knife while in her bathtub. In this, as in and many other similar situations, Comstock expressed no remorse, calling it a "bloody end to a bloody life." It is reported that she was the 15th individual he had driven to self-destruction. It was only in later life that Comstock ceased to brag of these suicides.

The details of Comstock's long campaigns against obscenity, pornography, and even consumption of alcohol need not concern us further. It is sufficient to say that the above pattern of entrapment was his modus operandi even to the point of persuading otherwise guiltless individuals into legal transgressions. In 1874, the heyday of his sanctimonious Armageddon against the purveyors of smut, the YMCA reported that he had seized 134,000 pounds of obscene books, 194,000 lewd pictures and photographs, 14,200 pounds of stereotype plates, 60,300 articles "made of rubber for immoral purposes," 5500 sets of playing cards, and 31,150 boxes of pills and powders, (mostly "aphrodisiacs"). In a 1913 interview, he boasted of having convicted enough people to fill a passenger train of 61 coaches.

Ultimately, by aiming at fewer and less flagrant offenders, his campaign caused a reaction. His condemnation of works of pictorial art based on mere nudity, his restrictions on works of literature such as James Joyce's "Ulysses," Henry Miller's "Tropic of Cancer," even the works of Sigmund Freud, fueled the flames of an incipient counterculture. Worse, he became the subject of mockery, the object of cartoons lampooning his appalling prudery. In one instance he is shown dragging backward, by the scruff of the neck, a supine young woman in her nightgown accusing her before a judge of having given birth to a naked infant.

Nevertheless, as late as 1915, he arrested Margaret Sanger's husband, Bill Sanger, and convicted him of possession of a pamphlet on birth control, "Family Limitation," written and published by his wife. An agent of the Society for the Suppression of Vice secured the evidence, and Sanger, despite his plea of being father and at that time sole parent to their three children, (Margaret was in Europe), was sentenced to jail for 30 days, which he served rather than pay the alternative of a fine of $150.

Finally, Comstock was relieved of his commission at the post office and even from his salaried position at the Society for the Suppression of Vice. President Wilson nevertheless appointed him to represent the Unites States at the Purity Congress at the San Francisco Exposition in July of 1915, but the train trip was hard on what was now an old man. Comstock became ill shortly upon his return. While attending the trial of William Sanger, he developed pneumonia and died quietly on the 21st of September. He was 71.

How is one to judge the Anthony Comstocks of this world? We must admire his energy in the relentless pursuit of his ideals, his incorruptibility, his unimpeachable personal morality, his compassion for and love of family. Yet here was a man who willingly stooped to the most debased means to entrap his quarries; a man who could shrug off their suicides and prolonged jail sentences as the justice of a righteous deity; a man incapable of contemplating an alternative view of society or of a human nature at variance with his own – ultimately a zealot of unassailable bigotry.

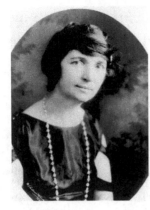

CHAPTER TWO

The Nurse
Margaret Louisa (Higgins) Sanger

"No woman is completely free unless she is wholly capable of controlling her fertility and ... no baby receives its full birthright unless it is born gleefully wanted by its parents."

Allan Guttmacher

A s a convenience, we will use the title of nurse to describe Margaret Sanger, for this was her stated profession and it was as such that she represented herself. We will ignore for the moment that she was never registered as a nurse in New York State, where she practiced, either under her maiden name or her married one, but recognizing that registration was not begun until December of 1903, one year after her nursing training terminated which indeed, she did not quite complete. This is not to detract from the monumental work she accomplished in pursuit of her goals and ideals, but simply to alert the reader to possible discrepancies in her biographies. Notwithstanding, she was a woman of energy, wit and political skill, who held strong convictions on the validity and rectitude of the causes she supported. One of these causes was the right of women to use birth control, a term she invented and a cause that led finally to the development of oral contraception. We use the term "women" advisedly, for at that time the only widely known methods of contraception were withdrawal and condoms, each of which was essentially a male option.

She was born on September 14th, 1879, in Corning, N.Y., the sixth of 11 children, and third of four daughters, to Irish immigrant parents. (Margaret later obfuscated her date of birth to make herself seem younger.) Her mother, Anne Purcell Higgins, was a devout Catholic who died of tuberculosis in 1899. Apart from giving birth to 11 children, Anne Higgins is said to have suffered seven spontaneous abortions. Margaret's father, Michael Hennessey Higgins, was a part-time stone mason who, in addition to his regular employment at the Corning Glass Works, made a sporadic if uncertain living from carving headstones. He played an important role in the 1890 strike against his employers. His independence of mind and political iconoclasm undoubtedly influenced his daughter's later stances on socialism and other views that were unconventional for the times. For example, he invited Robert Ingersoll, a notorious atheist, to give an address in Corning. The local priest locked up the church hall where Ingersoll was scheduled to speak, so that assembled crowd had to adjourn to an open-air location. This and other anti-religious forays did not endear him to the local Catholic Church.

In the working class milieu of Corning, the future of most young women was that of marriage to a factory employee of the local Corning Glass Works, but in the Higgins family, encouraged by their enlightened father, each child pursued an education. Rebellious by nature, Margaret walked out of school in eighth grade, refusing to return after an altercation with a churlish teacher who upbraided her for being two minutes late for class. This crisis in Margaret's education was saved by the intervention of her two older sisters, Mary and Anne (Nan) Higgins, who undertook to finance her high school education at Claverack College and Hudson River Institute, a small, private, liberal arts school that closed in 1902. Mary paid the modest fees while Nan bought Margaret's books. Even so, Margaret had to work for her room and board. There is little doubt that Margaret Sanger was both intelligent and physically attractive. At Claverack, she was remembered by Amelia Stewart, a fellow student and friend, as "one of the most popular girls in school, popular with both boys and girls." It is reported that she could cook, sew, and dance with proficiency. In addition she excelled at her class work without becoming a bookworm. It was at this high school that she displayed her early interest in women's suffrage by presenting and reading an essay to the assembled school on women's rights, which, not surprisingly, was met with the contumely of her male classmates.

High school education ended prematurely because of financial difficulties and her mother's terminal illness. It is significant that she returned home to nurse her mother until her death on 31st March, 1899, at the age of 50 from a long-standing tubercular condition. Clearly, multiple pregnancies with abortions and the responsibility for the care of 11 children were contributory, but it is also reported that Anne Higgins had cervical cancer, essentially a venereal disease. After her mother's death and a difficult year dealing with her father's angry grief compounded by the care of her younger siblings, Margaret entered nursing training in 1900 as a probationer at White Plains Hospital, a substitute for an ambition to enter medical school at Cornell, for which she sorely lacked academic qualification. Like much nursing training of the time and even much later, it tested her endurance to the limit. In a letter to her sister Mary, she describes her long working hours with little time for sleep. ("Now talk about work! I slept just four hours out of 74 – and about ten hours all last week.")[2]

During her training she developed a tuberculosis infection of her neck glands. She had two operations that left her with a sinus drainage of the surgical wound, a discharge that persisted for the next 20 years. (Some years later, around the time of her first pregnancy, this was complicated by pulmonary tuberculosis, for which she spent a year in a sanatorium near Saranac, N.Y., under the care of renowned specialist Edward Trudeau.) Her nursing training was terminated abruptly just weeks before completion by her precipitate marriage in 1902 to William Sanger, whom she met at an informal dance when she was a nursing intern at the Manhattan Eye and Ear Infirmary. In his letters to her, William Sanger describes with great optimism his career prospects as an architect and consequent financial security. William had arrived in New York at the age of 5, the son of German Jewish immigrants. Margaret often described the Sangers as well-to-do, but in fact they lived in a series of poor neighborhoods. Bill Sanger had had some architectural and art training at the Cooper Union in New York, but at the time of their marriage, it seems likely that he was unemployed. Nevertheless, he was later able to obtain sufficient commissions to afford the building of a house in the exclusive suburb of Hastings-on-Hudson, where they had first moved into a rental home. Started in 1908 and furbished with modern architectural design, it became something of a showplace. One major feature was a stained glass rose window overlooking the staircase that Margaret and Bill designed and painfully constructed over many months of labor. Alas, a furnace fire destroyed the home

---

2   Your author is no stranger to sleep deprivation and is skeptical of Margaret's assertions, considering it another of her obfuscations of the truth.

and the rose window, composed with such care, only days after the couple moved in. Restructuring left Bill with an overwhelming debt estimated in excess of $12,000. Margaret and her husband lived in the reconstructed home until 1910 where – apart from the above-mentioned bout of tubercular infection following the difficult delivery of the first of her three children – she lived an uneventful if chaotic life, for reputably she was neither a good housekeeper nor attentive mother. William, for a time, seems to have continued to make a comfortable living designing and building houses.

In 1910, the couple sold their rebuilt home, carrying back the mortgage, and moved into a working class area of Northern Manhattan. Bill Sanger had meantime developed radical ideas and become a member of the Socialist Party. He relinquished his profession of architecture to make a tenuous living as an artist. Economic strains pressured Margaret into returning to her work as a nurse, albeit with enthusiasm, having found suburban life dull compared with the life-and-death drama of her professional career. Her mother-in-law facilitated her employment by taking care of the children. There is little doubt that her work among the working class poor greatly influenced Margaret Sanger's views on multiple child-bearing, maternal death, and the option of contraception. In her autobiography, she describes with great poignancy her care in 1912 of a young woman dying from her second illegal abortion. She recounts the pleadings of her female patients for information on birth control, as if they felt that she, as a nurse, had an all-encompassing knowledge of such matters. In fact, as noted, only two methods of contraception were known at that time, condoms and withdrawal, each dependent on the uncertain motivation of the husband. Moreover, as we have seen, it was expressly forbidden by law even to discuss such matters. It was then that she "resolved…to do something to change the destinies of mothers whose miseries were as vast as the sky."

Both she and her husband became involved in socialist organizations, including the Industrial Workers of the World (IWW or, more colloquially, the Wobblies) a group without any reservations regarding the promotion of strikes or sabotage. Consistent with other Western nations, the American Industrial Revolution of the mid 1800s had brought appalling living and working conditions to the poor of the cities. Child labor was rife. Most adults, men and women alike, were forced into dismal labor or factory work for long hours, often without as much as a half-day off. People, accustomed to the relative freedom of farm labor and rural domesticity, were forced into crowded, unsanitary workplaces and dwellings with their consequences of ill health, disease, physical exhaustion and despair. Such a menial environment was ripe for socialist ideology. Its leaders looked with resentment at the wide disparity between the downtrodden workers and their wealthy capitalist masters. Strikes, sabotage, even assassination, were their weapons. Their propaganda was spread by pamphlets and left-leaning newspapers.

It was in 1911 that Margaret Sanger began writing a Sunday column for the New York Call. This publication, founded in 1908, soon established itself as the leading Socialist newspaper of the time until it closed down in 1923. Sanger's column was eventually titled "What Every Girl Should Know." Around May of 1912, when she proposed to write about venereal disease, the Call was notified by the post office that if it were to run such articles the entire issue would be suppressed. Instead of her two-column article, the newspaper, under the usual heading of "What Every Girl Should Know" printed in bold type the word, "NOTHING." This was Margaret's introduction to the Comstock laws.

She became involved indirectly in the famous January 1912 strike of the Lawrence, Mass. textile mills. Margaret was given responsibility for the evacuation to New York of the strikers' children. The 119 children were in pitiable condition – undernourished and poorly clad against the bitter cold of February. A congressional inquiry followed and there we see Margaret defending her actions before the Committee of Rules of the House of Representatives. Her testimony before a sympathetic group of legislators was clear, unhurried and factual with no hint of the anger she must have felt at the meager status of her charges. It is noteworthy that one of the sympathetic members of the audience was none other than Helen Taft, wife of William Howard Taft, president of the United States.

In April of 1913, Margaret participated in the silk mill strike in Hazelton, Pa. Along with 18 young women, she was incarcerated for five days in a filthy, unsanitary jail with limited toilet facilities and, for sustenance, two cups of water per day and a loaf of bread. Some of the free-love philosophies of the social and political contacts of the Sangers permitted her, at this time, to take at least one lover. From the spring of 1913 continuing through a summer vacation in Province-town, Mass., she had as one of her many paramours John Rompapas, a handsome anarchist she had met at the home of Mabel Dodge, the latter a wealthy socialite with liberal leanings. Not surprisingly her marriage became threatened, not least by the economic deprivation attendant upon Bill's avocation as an artist. Now the parents of three children, Grant, Stuart and Peggy, she and Bill left for Paris via Glasgow on October 16th, 1913, and Margaret enlightened herself on European methods and ideas on contraception, in particular the use of the contraceptive diaphragm, while Bill excitedly explored the work of French Impressionist artists.

As the marriage continued to fall apart, Margaret, after a month in Paris, returned to New York on 23rd December accompanied by their three children, leaving her husband in Paris to his artistic aspirations. Although Bill, to the end, was faithful to Margaret, sending her frequent, pathetic letters (mostly unanswered) professing his love, this marked the functional end of their marriage.

Upon return to New York, she rented a dingy flat and survived economically by some work in nursing and midwifery. She proposed publication of a paper that issued contraceptive advice, and received advance subscriptions from supporters including impoverished women desperate for such information. The first issue of The Woman Rebel was published in March of 1914. Its goals were multiple and ill-focused, but certainly one of them was the dissemination of information on contraception. The second issue provided a column on contraception without however, describing any method. Its tone was philosophical in content, exhorting women in general to consider the concept, advocating the overturn of restrictive laws.

Comstock, who had been keeping an eye on the publication, had it barred from the mails on tenuous legal grounds. Furious, Margaret responded with a series of virulent, wide-ranging, ill-focused diatribes on everything from women's rights to abortion, or as some called it, "rebellion for rebellion's sake." Inevitably this led to further suppression of the paper so that her subscribers, deprived of their promised information on contraception, began to complain. Finally, after her August issue, with its assault on the institution of marriage and childbearing and a particularly offensive article in defense of assassination written by radical free speech activist Herbert Thorpe, she was indicted for the publication of lewd and indecent articles, and with incitement to murder and riot. While awaiting trial, she wrote a pamphlet called "Family Limitation," describing different methods of birth control – some, incidentally, quite ineffective. With great difficulty she found a willing printer and distributed 100,000 copies. Brought to trial in October 1914 and with a one-week extension on bail raised by her friends, she peremptorily took train for Montreal and there, with a forged passport under the name of Bertha Watson, boarded ship for Liverpool, leaving her three children in the care of Bill Sanger, who had just returned from France.

The year spent in Great Britain, chiefly in London, had a great influence on Margaret Sanger. It provided her with time to study, preliminarily at the British Museum, and to form friendships with some of the more forward thinkers of contemporary British society, among whom was Havelock Ellis. Ellis was the shy, retiring, sexually constrained author of the seven-volume "Psychology of Sex," a work, because of its sexual context, available only to members of the medical profession until released for public consumption in 1935. Ellis became her mentor, advising her on her studies and directing her reading, encouraging her to focus on birth control to the exclusion of her interests in socialism and women's suffrage. Meantime, back in New York, Bill Sanger had been entrapped by none other than Comstock himself into selling to one of his agents a copy of "Family Limitation." He was arrested in January of 1915, but was not tried until the following September.

In February of 1915, with the encouragement of Ellis and financed by monies from the sale of her "Family Limitation" pamphlet, Margaret left for Holland with letters of introduction to doctors and midwives. Notwithstanding that Europe was deeply involved in World War I, she was easily able to travel on her American passport still under the name of Bertha Watson. From her readings, she had learned that in Holland there were advances in the use of the contraceptive diaphragm. Indeed, in 1883 a Dr. Wilhelm Mensinga of Flensburg, Germany, had published a description of such a device. This had been perfected with the cooperation of Dr. Aletta Jacobs (1854-1929) of Amsterdam, the first woman in the Netherlands to graduate from a medical school. Jacobs was the eighth of 12 children of a Jewish doctor. Margaret had learned through her studies that, within a five-mile radius of Dr. Jacobs' clinics serving the poor, the frequency and incidence of stillbirths, abortions and venereal disease had dropped. Jacobs, despite the success of her work, had had a most difficult time dealing with the criticisms not only of her male col-leagues, some at least envious of her professional success, but also of the clergy, many of whose wives had, ironically, been among her clientele.

Philosophically, Jacobs wrestled with the perceived potential consequences of contraception, for many argued that with ready availability, population would drop to "a world without children," and that adultery and promiscuity would increase. Thus, the idea of birth prevention had some unsavory connotations, some of which are still with us today. However, like Margaret Sanger, Aletta Jacobs "was haunted by the suffering caused by frequent pregnancies, which for various reasons, can have a disastrous effect on a woman's life."

It is recorded that Dr. Jacobs refused to meet with Margaret on the basis that she was a mere nurse. In fairness to the doctor, the connotation of nurse did not equate with the American profes-sion. In Dutch society, nurses were mere household help occasionally charged with looking after the sick. However, Margaret was warmly received by Dr. Johannes Rutgers, head of the Neo-Malthusian League. Malthusian philosophy saw the world population as doomed to eventual starvation from uncontrolled reproduction, an idea that still resonates today. However, he and his fellow league members were also cognizant of the miseries of uncontrolled fertility. Like his colleague Dr. Jacobs, Rutgers also had to deal with the pervasive criticism of his ideas. Although by this time he was quite elderly and had a limited knowledge of English, he did take Margaret to some of the clinics, where she was able to confer with midwives who were being instructed by Dr. Rutgers in the use of the diaphragm. She records that, notwithstanding the language difficulties, she herself was able to instruct 75 Dutch women in its use.

Curiously, despite the thousands of members of the Dutch Neo-Malthusian League, the presence of some 54 clinics, and the ready availability of contraceptive supplies in shops, many of the Dutch seemed unaware of these innovations. Small wonder then that news of these activities had reached neither Great Britain nor the United States.

Under difficult conditions due to the war and German submarine activities, Margaret was barely able to persuade a ship's captain to make an exception of her, a woman, and include her on a hazardous trip across the English Channel back to London. By this time, she had concluded that dissemination of birth control information would take more than pamphlets, talks or books, but would require the adoption of the Dutch techniques of clinics staffed by trained personnel, be they doctors, midwives or nurses. Via Paris, Margaret traveled to Barcelona to join one of her many lovers, the Spanish revolutionary and teacher Lorenzo Portet, whom she had met in Liverpool almost immediately upon her arrival in England in November of 1914. She sojourned with him over an idyllic three months before returning to England in April of 1915 while Portet returned to his publishing business in Paris. It is a curious commentary on their relationship that Portet's wife and family were resident in Barcelona at the same time.

Meantime, events on the other side of the Atlantic were eclipsing Margaret Sanger's leadership. Bill Sanger was finally brought to trial in 1915 and sentenced to a month in prison from 10th September through 9th October after refusing the alternative of a $150 fine. The trial, before Judge James McInerney, a man of devout Catholic persuasion, was accompanied by the loud demonstrations of Sanger's supporters. Incidentally, Comstock, who had attended the trial in person and heatedly denounced Sanger's supporters, shortly took ill of pneumonia and died later that month, a fact foreseen to be of some assistance in Margaret's own upcoming trial although of course, his laws were still extant.

To her anger and irritation, Margaret had learned that the momentum of the birth control movement had been taken over by the formation of the National Birth Control League under the leadership of Mary Ware Dennett with the assistance of Anita Block, editor of the Call, and was now financed in part by the wealthy socialite Clara Stillman. Feeling that events were passing her by, at the end of September she set sail from Bordeaux, arriving in New York on 6th October, a few days before Bill's release from jail. Although received warmly by the officers of National Birth Control League, she quickly learned that philosophically they were disposed to change the law rather than to defy it and they refused her any financial support.

It was at this time that Margaret experienced one of life's greatest tragedies, the death of a child. During her stay abroad, Stuart, Grant and Peggy had been variously under the care of Bill and of friends and relatives. They had spent much of the time at a variety of boarding schools, some of doubtful worth. Peggy, who had contracted polio at an early age, developed pneumonia. She was admitted to Mt. Sinai hospital, where Margaret's younger sister, Ethel Byrne, a staff nurse, gave her personal care. But Peggy, only 5 years old, died within days of admission on 6th November. Margaret was devastated, for Peggy had been her favorite. For the rest of her life, she mourned on the anniversary of the child's death.

And now Margaret Sanger was faced with her long-delayed trial, charged as she was with sending obscene material through the United States mail. Although the law had technically been broken, the weakness of the government's case and the wave of public sympathy for Margaret compounded by the death of Peggy resulted in powerful popular and financial support for her cause. Had she entered a plea of guilty with a promise not to break the law in future, it would have resulted in exoneration, but Sanger, despite the advice of close friends and lawyers to accept, wanted a jury trial with its attendant publicity. The New York Sun commented that the situation ironically "presents the anomaly of a prosecutor loath to prosecute and a defendant anxious to be tried." The trial was finally set for 24th January, 1916, but in response to the adverse publicity, the judge adjourned the case for a week. On 18th February the government entered a "nolle prosequi" depriving Margaret of her much-wanted publicity. The result led to confirmation of her belief that the furtherance of her cause could not be obtained by the publication of pamphlets and the written word, but rather by defiance of the law and by opening clinics in the manner of those she had seen and experienced in Holland.

During the spring and summer of 1916 she embarked on an exhausting lecture tour, which took her to most of the major cities of the United States. Although she was arrested in Portland, Ore., and put in jail overnight with three other women, in general, not only were her lectures were well received, but at times with great enthusiasm. In addition, they generated financial support not only from wealthy liberal matrons, but also from many subscribers of lesser means. Upon her return to New York on or around 16th July, she publicly announced her intention of opening a birth control clinic.

An enterprise such as this was quite clearly illegal. Section 1142 of the New York statutes forbade anyone from giving out contraceptive information to anybody for any reason. Paradoxically, section 1145 of the same statutes specifically enabled physicians to write prescriptions for the prevention of conception or to prevent disease. Margaret planned to challenge the law with the hope that the attendant publicity of her cause would lead, if not to abrogation of the law, at least to an increase in the social acceptance of birth control.

We might pause here to review her philosophy and motivation for the concept of birth control. Apart from simple freedom of choice, it was bound up with the eugenic theories of the time so that contraception was advocated by the Neo-Malthusians for those with diseases that were transmissible or at least thought to be so, on the basis of contemporary knowledge. Syphilis and gonorrhea, certainly known to be transmissible to the fetus, insanity less so, and epilepsy hardly at all, were included in her recommendations for birth control. Physical illness of the mother, either detrimental to the pregnancy or vice versa, was also included; for example, diseases of the heart, lungs or kidneys. She advocated delayed pregnancy until the couple were in their 20s, still today regarded as the optimal time for childbearing both from the point of view of the safety of the mother and for the well-being of the fetus. Contraception was also recommended for purely economic considerations based on family income and the number of children already on scene. As a final recommendation, she advised the spacing of childbirth by two to three years. Sanger, with profound socialist convictions, felt too, that indiscriminate reproduction fed the capitalist system with a constant supply of cheap labor and that this constituted the rationale for much of government and legislative resistance to change.

Many of these principles still carry weight today, although eugenic theories of that time have been looked at askance in the light of modern knowledge of heredity. Even so, the modern science of genetics has lent greater accuracy in the prediction of physical, mental or metabolic disease in offspring, always with the freedom of the parents or prospective parents as to independent action.

Unable to locate a willing doctor to work in her putative clinic, Margaret determined to go ahead with the assistance of her sister Ethel Byrne, a registered nurse. A chance meeting with five distressed and fertile mothers from the Brownsville section of Brooklyn persuaded her in that geographic direction. A certain Mr. Rabinowitz, a property owner sympathetic to her goals, proved willing to lease 46 Amboy St. at the low rate of $50 per month, a sum that Margaret had just received from a woman in Los Angeles in support of her cause. Without ever receiving a reply, Margaret wrote an "in your face" letter to the Brooklyn district attorney advising him of her intentions. She planned only to show cervical pessaries to her clientele and tell them of the principles of contraception. According to her autobiography, on the morning of the 16th October, 1916, she opened the "first birth control clinic in America." She reports that on the first day, about 150 women lined up at the door. She and Ethel worked until 7 that evening until they could work no more, asking the remaining women to return the next day.

It was not long before the clinic attracted the attention of the law. A policewoman, purporting to be a client, came for advice and returned the next day with a warrant for their arrest. Rather than ride in the police wagon, Margaret insisted on walking the mile distance to the courthouse, where she and Ethel were ordered to the Raymond Street Jail, a cold, filthy, malodorous, vermin-infested prison. Released the next day, she returned to the clinic only to find that the police had forced her landlord, Mr. Rabinowitz to sign eviction papers.

Ethel Byrne, her sister, was the first to be tried on 8th January, 1917. Inevitably she was found guilty of violating Section 1142 of the New York Statutes, which made it illegal to give out contraceptive information. Margaret was naively convinced that if she were allowed to state the logic of her case in court, she and her fellows would be discharged. Alas, just like anybody, she was faced with the technical realities of the law. The court was neither obliged to hear nor even interested in any personal defense. Ethel was sentenced to 30 days in the workhouse of the notorious Blackwell Prison, where she immediately went on a hunger strike, refusing not only food but also water. After three days, in an assault without precedent in the annals of American prisons, she was force-fed. Her resistance resulted in a year of physical impairment and convalescence. Nevertheless, during her incarceration, day-to-day reports on her condition caused widespread discussion in the press and among readers.

Margaret was scheduled for trial on 29th January, along with the clinic secretary, Fania Mindell, who was accused of distributing copies of "What Every Girl Should Know." Fania was found guilty and fined $50. It was inevitable that the court would find Margaret guilty as charged. Her refusal to promise future compliance with the law before a sympathetic court that was willing, given this undertaking, to exonerate her, led to a sentence of 30 days in the workhouse. She was incarcerated in Queens Penitentiary from the 4th February until the 6th March. In contrast to her previous experiences, she enjoyed considerable latitude during her imprisonment. She and fellow prisoners were not put behind bars, but had each a small alcove for a bed, toilet and washstand. The matron, a coarse but not unkindly woman, allowed her freedom from work, permitting her to write at leisure and to teach reading to some of the illiterate inmates. Margaret's only revolt was her physical resistance to any attempt at fingerprinting her like a common criminal. In this she was successful.

Once released, she began publishing the magazine Birth Control Review. She also began a long love affair with her defense lawyer, Josiah Goldstein. The magazine never did, and legally could not, disclose specific information on methods of contraception, despite the written pleas of many of its readers. (Even at this time, one of Margaret's employees, Kitty Marion was entrapped by a member of the Society for the Suppression of Vice into giving out information on birth control and was given a jail sentence.) Instead, the magazine focused on the philosophical, political and legal aspects of the controversy. With some interruptions it continued publication over the next four years and became a source of badly needed income. In addition, it provided Margaret with the needed publicity for her cause. Even so, no newsstand would carry the magazine, so that it had to be sold on the street by individual volunteers or by subscription. She formed the New York Birth Control League hiring a savvy treasurer, Frederick Blossom. Inevitably this led to competition with

Mary Dennett's National Birth Control League. One of Margaret's characteristics was that she would brook no competition for leadership of her cause. Another example of this was her later quarrel with Blossom, whose organizational abilities and expertise in fundraising became a similar threat. Margaret set up headquarters in an office at 104 Fifth Avenue. On the door was the insignia Birth Control. With the help of her sister Ethel Byrne and a 17-year-old loyal secretary, Anna Lifshiz, she continued to distribute her pamphlet, Family Limitation. To avoid confrontation with the law, the material was mailed to recipients from various locations throughout the city so that the senders could not be traced. It is recorded that she had 200 to 300 requests per day for this publication. In January of 1918, her lover and lawyer, Josiah Goldstein won a significant legal victory by getting the New York Court of Appeals declare that information on contraception, which could be given legally to males for prevention of disease, could now be given to females for the same purpose. Although this provided her with the opportunity of opening a birth control clinic, Margaret did not follow through, probably because of lack of funds.

Later in 1918 she had surgery for her tubercular glands. During her convalescence, she began writing a book titled "Woman and the New Race." Unlike her former diatribes in "The Woman Rebel," this was more dispassionate, citing statistics and other supportive arguments in favor of birth control. Besides the more obvious economic rationale for the use of birth control by poor but fecund women, the tract was interlaced with eugenic theories on reducing the reproduction of the feeble-minded as well as current socialist dogma about reducing the production of "wage slaves."

In February of 1919, tired of her lecture circuit, she left by train for California accompanied by Grant, her younger and more withdrawn son. Although she gave several well-attended lectures, she became despondent over the reported death from tuberculosis of her former lover Portet and the written importunities of Josiah Goldstein requesting that she marry him. Torn between her affection for him and her burning desire for independence, she was reduced at times to tears. Nevertheless, shortly she embarked for England, where she renewed her friendship with Havelock Ellis and was introduced to H.G. Wells, soon to become yet another of her lovers. But meantime, even as she continued on a lecture tour of Great Britain, she fell in love with a handsome, educated, upper-class Englishman, Hugh de Selincourt, who shared her enthusiasm for poetry.

In 1920, Margaret Sanger again visited Great Britain and Ireland, consorting with such greats as H.G. Wells, with whom she had an affair despite his marriage to his vivacious second wife, Amy Catherine, whom he called Jane. Jane either did not care or simply chose to ignore the liaison. Once more, Margaret gave a series of lectures up and down the country, the populace now more receptive to her ideas after the publication of "Married Love" by Marie Stopes, its brilliant but strange British author. Marie Stopes was yet another with whom Margaret quarreled over the threat of leadership of the birth control movement. She also spent time with Havelock Ellis, on a tour of Ireland.

By 1921, Margaret was back in New York, where she met Noah Slee, the man who would become her second husband. The relationship was one only a cynic could love. Her first recorded meeting with him was at a dinner date on 5th April, 1921. Slee's personality was a contrast to Margaret's. A stolid, overweight, balding man in his mid-60s he had been born in Capetown, South Africa, the grandson of an Episcopal minister. His great saving grace was a fortune reckoned at around $9 million. Rising from a penniless boyhood, he had earned his money by shrewd investments and the sale of his Three-in-One Oil company, a product used in the lubrication of bicycle chains. There were a couple of impediments to their later marriage – their current spouses! Margaret was long estranged from Bill Sanger. However it seems that she went through the formality of a divorce in October of 1921. She did not formally advise anybody including Bill Sanger of this legality fearing, as a birth control advocate, the additional critical opposition of the Catholic Church once it was learned that she was a divorcee. Slee was still married to his socially well-connected but quite frigid wife. Obviously for him, marriage to an attractive, witty and much younger wife had its allure, but for Margaret the chief attraction of the prospective union was that it would afford her the money she needed to further her goals. She had long dreamed of finding a rich widower as a husband. Even before their marriage, Slee became a devoted supporter of her cause, supplying her with business advice and financial support.

She returned to New York in November of 1921, set on planning a conference on birth control. This was to be the First American Birth Control Conference held at the Plaza Hotel. On the third day of the three-day conference, the capacious auditorium of Town Hall on 42nd Street was rented for her public presentation on "Birth Control! Is it Moral?" Accompanied by old friends Juliet Rublee, a wealthy socialite, and Harold Cox, a former member of Parliament in the British government and editor of the Edinburgh Review, she arrived at the auditorium only to find the entrance barred by members of the New York Police Department. Ducking through another entry way, Margaret was still prevented from addressing the audience. It was learned during the confrontation with the police that the meeting had been ordered closed by none other than the Archbishop of New York, Patrick Hayes, clearly without any legal authority to do so. In the turmoil, Margaret was able to manipulate the police into arresting her along with Juliet and two other women friends. They were immediately released pending a morning court appearance. As a result, Margaret won a tremendous public relations victory. The news reached the newspapers, which responded with the expected diatribes on the abuse of free speech. The attendant publicity continued for weeks, during which time there were two inconclusive investigations as to the source of the orders given to the police force. The name of Margaret Sanger, hitherto relatively obscure, now became known ubiquitously. As an addendum, it should be noted that just a few days before the conference, Margaret Sanger, conferring with her friends, formed the American Birth Control League. Its aims were to further information on, and provide access to, birth control.

The action of Archbishop Hayes in closing off the conference was one of breathtaking arrogance. With no legal authority what-soever, he, as the leader of a minority sect in a country whose con-stitution specifically contravened the establishment of an organized religion, used his power and influence to abuse the constitutional rights of freedom of speech and peaceable assembly. It is of interest to record his rationale, revealed in his Christmas pastorale:

"Children troop down from Heaven because God wills it. He alone has the right to stay their coming; while he blesses some homes with many, others with few, or with none at all. They come in the way ordained by his wisdom. Woe to them who degrade, pervert or do violence to that law of nature as fixed by the eternal decree of God himself. Even though some little angels in the flesh, through moral, mental or physical deformity of the parents may appear to human eyes as misshapen, a blot on civilized society, we must not lose sight of this Christian thought that under and with this visible malformation there lives the immortal soul to be saved and glorified for all eternity among the blessed in Heaven."

In February of 1922 Margaret embarked on an Asian lecture tour that included Japan, Korea and China. She was accompanied by her second son, Grant, and Noah Slee, but her diary of the time scarcely denotes the presence of the latter, although it seems that he did underwrite her expenses. Her trip ended in England, where she attended the Fifth International Neo-Malthusian Conference in London, acting as chair of one of the sessions and reporting to a sympathetic audience her Asian experiences. Despite the romantic overtures of Noah, she renewed her liaison with Hugh de Selincourt, besides having a brief fling with H.G. Wells. Noah's whereabouts during this time are uncertain, but quite suddenly and secretively she and Slee were married in a registrar's office in London on 18th September, 1922, Slee having secured an August divorce in Paris from his American wife. As noted, their marriage was a most unlikely union. First, she had just turned 42, while Slee was 20 years her senior. His religious piety was in stark contrast to Margaret's rampant atheism, while his punctiliousness and cautious business-like approach to life was a counterpoint to her rebellious outlook and undisciplined philosophy. He contributed generously of his time and money, and of his business and manufacturing expertise in the promotion of her cause. But his ardent desire for her affection and her need for financial support and experienced counsel made for a satisfactory working relationship that somehow survived Margaret's demands for separate residencies, each with its own key for access. Nevertheless,

Margaret continued to engage in a series of casual sexual affairs, of which Slee was either unaware or pretended ignorance.

Once back in New York, Slee refused to fund Margaret's ambition to open a clinic. However, out of the blue, wealthy Englishman Clinton Chance responded to her telegraphed appeal with $5,000, enough to cover the salary of a physician, Dr. Dorothy Bocker. This was a large salary in those days, but was necessary to compensate Dorothy Bocker for her move from a safe employment situation in Georgia and the risk of her arrest and imprisonment in New York. In addition, Clinton Chance paid for the necessary equipment of the office and examining room. With Goldstein's legal victory of January 1918, it was now possible for doctors to give contraceptive advice to women for health reasons, so the facility was termed a Research Clinic avoiding the term birth control. Each client had to be documented as to the specific health condition that merited birth control, although without question these conditions were extended from the absolute to the tenuous. The clientele were fitted with Dutch caps – or diaphragms – a covering of the uterine cervix. However, of 2,700 applicants, only 900 qualified for "health reasons," the only condition that would satisfy the law. These contraceptive items were not only illegal, but also expensive, and had to be smuggled into the country from Holland. A friendly Italian coal merchant who was also a rum runner offered help and, with the assistance of Noah Slee who agreed to ship diaphragms to just outside the 12-mile offshore limit, the clinic soon had a safe supply. In addition, Slee shipped large numbers to Montreal, later smuggling them over the U.S.-Canadian border. Later, Slee, recognizing a real estate bargain, enabled Margaret to move the clinic to a more substantial building that he had purchased for that purpose.

Meantime Dr. Bocker declined to continue working after the expiration of her two-year contract. Not for the first time, Margaret had proven imperial and authoritative. Bocker's resignation worked to Margaret's advantage, for she was able to substitute Dr. Hannah Stone, whose husband, Dr. Abraham Stone, was not only a noted gynecologist but was also the editor of a respected journal on infertility. In addition, Dr. Hannah Stone not only proved assiduous in her work, carefully documenting and conserving patient data, but also volunteered to work without salary. Through this couple, Margaret hoped to influence the medical establishment to support her cause. Somewhat later, with money supplied by her husband, she was able to secure as medical director the esteemed Dr. James Cooper, a zealous supporter of birth control.

In 1925, a second office of the so-named Clinical Research Bureau opened at 46 W. 15th Street. Without interference from the law, the clinic continued until April 15, 1929, when police raided it. A policewoman, Anna McNamara, posing as a client, received contraceptive advice, which served as the rationale. The raid was directed by Mrs. Mary Sullivan of the New York Police Department, head of the City Policewoman's Bureau who was there in person to supervise. In their indiscriminate haste, the police, in addition to seizing contraceptive devices and much irrelevant material, also purloined patients' confidential records.

The medical profession was outraged, not so much by the raid as by the seizure of medical records, the confidentiality of which were, and still are, deemed sacrosanct. Consequently, the New York Medical Society passed a resolution protesting the action. Now, not only did Margaret have publicity, which led to a sharp upsurge in clinic attendance, but she also had fortuitously gained the formal alliance of the medical profession. Further, she had confirmed the right of physicians to prescribe methods of birth control in the interests of the health of their female patients as supported by Section 1145 of the New York statutes despite the conflicting, all-encompassing Section 1142, which specifically forbade the dissemination of any contraceptive information by anyone for any reason.

In the years from 1925 to 1929, Margaret was far from idle. In March of 1925 she organized the meeting of the Sixth International Malthusian and Birth Control organization in New York, arranging for several prominent speakers from a variety of European countries, among whom was the Dutch doctor Aletta Jacobs, now more insightful and supportive of Sanger's work. It is interesting to note that the speakers were prevented by U.S law from discussing any specific method of birth control, but were confined to debating its philosophic values and demographic effects. This was baffling, even astonishing, to some of the European speakers, in whose countries debates on the topic were much more open and hardly subject to legal constraints.

A second international conference followed in the fall of 1927 in Geneva, an attractive location, for it was also the site of the headquarters of the League of Nations, thus affording Sanger the possibility of further publicity. She also hoped to co-opt the League into support of her principles. Incidentally, the reception and dinner for the speakers was held at the Chateau de Prangins at nearby Nyons, owned by Katharine McCormick, who donated the facility for that purpose. We will hear more of Mrs. McCormick later. By this time, the idea of birth control was out in the open but no less controversial. The debates were not so much on women's rights as on eugenics. The philosophy and theories of the time included limitation of procreation of the unfit and the promotion of larger families by the better-educated who were also (presumably) better-endowed genetically. Sanger also had to deal with the policies of the dictatorial governments of Japan, Italy and Germany, whose opposition to birth control was based on their goals of increasing population. Indeed, these governments were providing childbearing incentives such as medals, financial support and offers of property. This was happening despite the background of a rapid rise in world population, which had doubled between 1800 and 1900. This had become a source of international concern, a seeming confirmation of Malthusian theory, which declared that, ultimately, population growth would exceed the food supply necessary for its support.

Slowly, the idea of birth control was becoming accepted. Most significantly, the Lambeth conference of Anglican bishops in England in 1930, an event held at 10-year intervals, gave its approval to contraception. In 1934, the bishops of the American Episcopal Church reversed their opposition. Jewish rabbinical leaders adopted support, as did the Methodist Church. But the Catholic Church remained, and to this date still remains, adamantly opposed. In a December 1930 declaration Pope Pius XI issued the encyclical Casti Connubi (On Christian Marriage) reaffirming the Catholic Church's traditional stance of prohibiting artificial means of contraception. Paradoxically, at least to some logicians, the Church interpreted the use of rhythm as morally acceptable.

For a while, Margaret Sanger had attempted to overturn the Comstock Laws, but in 1931, she began to pay more attention to this strategy. Her rival, Mary Ware Dennett, leader of the Voluntary Parenthood League, had made unsuccessful attempts in this regard using as her rationale the right of free speech. Margaret however, thought the best approach was to enlist the help of the medical profession, rather than pursue public access to methods of birth control, which might lead to methods that were untried or improperly supervised as to quality. An invitation was extended to H.G. Wells to speak at a fund-raiser at the new Waldorf Astoria, which he, although averse to public speaking, accepted. The monies raised enabled Margaret to establish a National Committee on Federal Legislation for Birth Control with an office in Washington. In the late '20s and early '30s, Margaret and her supporters made many attempts at introducing congressional legislation, Despite assiduous attention to the enlightenment of congressmen and senators and the support of such leading lights as Dr. John Williams, obstetrician-in-chief at Johns Hopkins and author of what is still today, the definitive textbook on obstetrics, her initiatives were lost or voted down in committees. At one committee hearing, for example, her bill was voted down by a senator who had not even attended. Another vote died in committee in part due to the opposition of Father Charles Coughlin, a noted Detroit radio broadcaster, notorious racist, and staunch supporter of the tenets of the Catholic Church.

Almost forgotten in the legal struggle were attempts at practical assaults in testing the Comstock laws. Following an international conference that she sponsored in Zurich in 1930, Margaret had ordered importation of Japanese pessaries, which had been displayed at the conference. Customs officials seized and destroyed them. Not to be outdone, Margaret ordered a second shipment addressed to Dr. Hannah Stone, the physician director of the Clinical Research Clinic. It was her contention that legal grounds had been established that these could not be impounded when prescribed by a doctor for patients whose health, in the judgment of the physician, required contraceptive innovation. This shipment was also seized. Suit was filed in the name of Dr. Stone but not until 1935 did the case come before Judge Grover Moscowitz of the Federal District Court of Southern New York Margaret Sanger's case was argued successfully by a bright young lawyer, Morris Ernst. This was the same lawyer who had defended Margaret and her colleagues after the police raid of her clinic in April of '29. While the law seemingly forbade importation, in the legal opinion of Judge Moscowitz, the law was open to a more liberal interpretation permitting the importations. The government immediately appealed the decision to the Circuit Court of Appeals before Judges Augustus Hand, Learned Hand and Thomas Swan, who in the fall of 1936 upheld the Moscowitz decision. The government had the right of appeal, but such was the prestige of the deciding judges of the Appeals Court that none was filed. With commendable alacrity, Customs withdrew its embargo. The Moscowitz decision further clarified the hitherto uncertain right of a physician to prescribe contraceptives for protection of health but also to import contraceptive devices and send them through the mail without fear of legal intervention. While the court edict applied only to New York, Connecticut and Vermont, here was a landmark decision indeed. In the following year, the American Medical Association reversed its longstanding opposition. Thus was the principle of contraception finally accepted.

The importance of Margaret Sanger's work was that she finally made contraception, within certain confines, at last quite legal. One can look critically at her life, her dissembling on her age and other matters, her controversial love life, and egocentricity, but here was a woman of intelligence and spirit, willing to go to jail for her beliefs, beliefs that women should be relieved from the burden of unwanted pregnancies and childbearing and their detrimental social and health consequences; a woman willing to go to jail for her principles – and not jail in the modern sense, but to some of the most unsanitary, degrading confines imaginable.

By the mid 1930s, her written works and her organization of professional meetings and conventions had led to a wide degree of social acceptance. While the topic of birth control remained controversial and the subject of much debate, by now the arguments were out in the open. No doubt history was on her side, but without her leadership, intelligence, and tenacity these changes would have been much longer in coming.

While the principle of acceptance was established, the methods available were still not widely publicized. The only effective contraceptive for women remained the diaphragm. Still widely prescribed to this day, it has a fail rate of around 4%. It requires that the individual be fitted according to size and that the size be reviewed following childbirth or significant changes in weight. It has to be checked at different time intervals for deterioration or damage to its component rubber. However, it is without significant side effects. The search continued for a more effective method, one that could be separated from the sex act itself, and it is to this that we must now turn our attention.

CHAPTER THREE

Physiology

This chapter may be skipped by the less-intent reader, but in order to understand the mechanism of action of the oral contraceptive pill, some knowledge of the female reproductive system is in order.

At the vault of the vagina lies the uterus, or womb. The neck, or cervix, of the uterus protrudes into the vagina for about ½ inch. It may easily be felt either by self-examination or on pelvic examination by a physician or interested layperson. It has a firm texture often compared to the sensation of touching the end of one's nose. It is an intrinsic part of the uterus entirely congruent with its structure. It is penetrated by a narrow cervical canal, which permits the outflow of menstrual blood or the inflow of spermatozoa. In shape, the uterus resembles an upside down flattened pear of small size. The uterus is lined by the endometrium, likened to a soft, thin skin. This endometrium increases in thickness during the menstrual or monthly cycle, preparing for the nidation, or implantation, of a fertilized egg. It is largely cast off by menstruation, but after menstruation it again grows steadily thicker. After production of an egg by the ovary, which is called ovulation, the lining produces certain secretions thought to nourish a fertilized egg before it can secure its own blood supply from the formation of the placenta or afterbirth.

On either side of the top of the uterus extend the fallopian tubes, or salpinges. These are quite narrow, fragile structures of about three to six inches in length, freely mobile within the female pelvis. Their most distant ends are close, but not attached to, the ovaries. The ovaries are about the size and shape of the most distal segment of an adult thumb and are a pale grey in color.

The monthly menstrual cycle is under hormonal control. Hormones are relatively simple messenger chemicals produced by the body's endocrine glands. These include the thyroid gland in the neck, the adrenal glands located at the upper poles of the kidneys, and the so-called gonads (ovaries in the female and testes in the male). The endocrine glands are under the control of a master endocrine gland at the base of the brain called the pituitary, which produces for example, thyroid stimulating hormone (TSH for short), and adrenocorticotropic hormone, or ACTH. For control of the ovary, the pituitary produces not one but two hormones. The first of these is called follicular stimulating hormone, or FSH, and the second is called luteinising hormone, or LH. At birth, each ovary contains its full complement of eggs, estimated at around 300,000-400,000 in number. Once a woman reaches puberty, each month one of these eggs matures under the influence of FSH, which is produced at the beginning of the menstrual cycle. The egg is surrounded by an increasing number of cells that develop and enclose a small fluid-like cyst called a graafian follicle, in which the egg is contained. In addition, the FSH stimulates the ovary, via the graafian follicle to increase production of the essential female hormone, estrogen, which, besides being responsible for the changes of puberty, such as breast enlargement and the growth of pubic hair, is also each month responsible for the growth of the uterine lining or endometrium. As the level of estrogen rises in the bloodstream and with the approach of the middle of the month, the pituitary releases LH, which not only causes release of the egg from the ovary by rupture of the graafian follicle, but also causes the area from which the egg is released to produce a second hormone called progesterone. This collection of cells that surrounded the egg, or ova, is called a corpus luteum, meaning "yellow body," from its color. It is important to realize that this formation of the corpus luteum and its production of progesterone is common to all mammals. Progesterone causes further thickening of the uterine lining and the production of secretions from that lining in preparation for fertilization. Should, fertilization not occur, pituitary stimulation of ovarian hormone production ceases. The uterine lining is cast off with some loss of blood, which is perceived as menstruation. The egg, too, is flushed out, but is quite tiny and only barely visible to the naked eye.

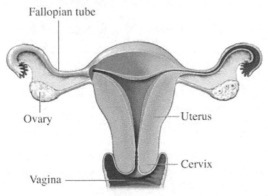

The ovarian hormones estrogen and progesterone are chemically quite similar in structure, although different in their effects. Indeed, they are little different from the male hormone testosterone or the adrenal hormone, cortisone. Collectively, these hormones are known as steroids, although the term has in recent years become associated with the illegal enhancement of athletic performance.

As we review the response of the pituitary to the rising level of estrogen causing it to release LH, it becomes apparent that if one could deceive the pituitary into thinking that egg production had taken place by administration of progesterone either by injection or by mouth, then it would not produce LH and ovulation would not take place. This is the basis of chemical contraception or the use of the birth control pill.

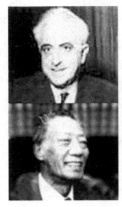

CHAPTER FOUR

The Biologists
Dr. Gregory Pincus
Dr. Min Chueh Chang

I t is important to realize from the outset that Dr. Gregory Pincus was not a physician. He was a biologist who performed his research mainly on rabbits and rats. This is not to derogate him, but to alert the reader to a major handicap in his research. That is to say, that although he was completely free to use drugs and medications on laboratory animals, he was not able to conduct drug trials on human subjects without the cooperation of a physician.

His close research associate was Min Chueh Chang who, in the annals of the history of the development of the birth control pill, is little-recognized outside the scientific community. His voluminous research was essentially on the fertilization of animal ovae, or eggs, by sperm, chiefly in rabbits and rats. Of his 347 publications, only a minimal number, five in all, were devoted to the observation of inhibition of ovulation, chiefly in rabbits and rats, by the administration of progesterone and progesterone-like steroids, but these were crucial to the development of the birth control pill.

Chang was born in Tai Yuan in the Shanxi province of China in 1908. His father, a magistrate, provided him with a university education in Peking (Beijing), where he graduated in 1933 with a degree in animal psychology. In 1938 he won a merit scholarship for study abroad and chose the field of agriculture at the University of Edinburgh. It is not surprising that he found the Scottish climate inhospitable, nor should it raise any eyebrows that he was not warmly received. Scotland, at that time, was essentially a closed ethnic culture. Foreigners, particularly Asians, had a difficult time assimilating. At the end of a year, he accepted an invitation to work on research at Cambridge. There he began his lifetime work on the biology of sperm, at first on rams, but later mostly on rabbits. The work on sheep should occasion little surprise, for these were the years of World War II food shortages (1939-45) and the British were interested in furthering meat production from this source. At Cambridge, Chang earned his Ph.D. in 1941

Gregory Pincus had worked at Cambridge before the war. On a later visit to Cambridge he met with Chang and invited him to join him in the United States, offering him a fellowship. In his autobiographical notes, Chang expresses his delight at the offer, for at Cambridge such a fellowship carried a lifetime income. (As we shall see, such was not the case in America.) With the post-war civil unrest in China, return was an unattractive proposition, so Chang accepted Pincus' offer and in 1945 went to work with him at the grandiloquently named Worcester Foundation for Experimental Biology in Shrewsbury, Mass. Later, he recalled, laughing in retrospection, that during the first year, research funding was in such short supply that he worked as a night watchman. Pincus was in California at the time of Chang's arrival, and Chang was met by Hudson Hoagland. The latter had set up a visiting professorship for Pincus at nearby Clark

University after Pincus had been passed over for promotion at Harvard. Hoagland at the time was busy with his own research in schizophrenia and when Chang presented himself at the hospital where Hoagland worked, he was at first mistaken for one of the patients!

Chang is reported as being tall and slim with a friendly personality and a rich sense of humor. Reportedly, his repartee would cause his audiences to erupt in uproarious bursts of laughter. His background of Confucianism had prepared him for a life of dedication to scientific enquiry. Indeed the volume of his work precluded all but a very slight interest in his family, which consisted of his wife, an American-born Chinese woman called Isabelle Chin, two daughters, and one son. Nor did he have any intellectual pursuits outside his work. Largely through the devotion of his wife, who shielded him from day-to-day family problems, he was able to work without domestic distractions and yet still commanded the respect and affection of his children. He and Greg Pincus developed a strong working relationship. While Chang's personality and growing reputation attracted a talented group of fellow researchers, he allowed them to work more or less independently, and many went on to establish their own excellent reputations in the field of mammalian reproduction. Chang performed pioneering work on in vitro fertilization in mammals. It was this research that ultimately led to the birth of Louise Joy Brown in Oldham, England, in 1978, the first successful result of human in vitro fertilization, reported by Patrick Steptoe, Bravister and Edwards. It was only later in Chang's career, and almost as a side interest, that at the urging of Pincus he conducted research on oral steroid contraception in mammals. As we have noted, these constituted a mere five publications out of his large repertoire and were published between 1951 and 1956. Founded at first on a shoestring budget, Chang's work in cooperation with Pincus ultimately resulted in the Worcester Foundation for Experimental Biology becoming a prominent and reputable research center. The volume and quality of Chang's research resulted in many awards, including an Albert Lasker award in 1954.

Gregory Goodwin ("Goody") Pincus was born to Russian Jewish immigrants on April 9, 1903, in Woodbine, NJ. His father, Joseph William Pincus was a teacher, editor of the Jewish Farmer, and an agricultural consultant. Gregory Pincus' undergraduate education took place at Cornell where he majored in pomology, or the study of apples. His ambition at the time was to have a career in agriculture. Moving from an interest in plant genetics to animal genetics, he undertook graduate studies at Harvard, receiving his doctorate in 1927. It was during this time that he met with Hudson Hoagland, whose career was destined to become inextricably meshed with his. Hoagland had graduated from Columbia and had gone on to earn an MS in chemical engineering at MIT. He continued his studies at Harvard, finishing in the same year as Pincus with a Ph.D. in experimental psychology; each received National Research Council Fellowships for post-doctoral work. Pincus chose to go to Cambridge University in England, where he began his interest in the physiology of reproduction. After a year and a half at Cambridge, he spent another 18 months at the Kaiser Wilhelm Institute in Berlin, returning to Harvard in 1930 as an instructor in the department of physiology where, in 1932, he was given a three- year appointment as assistant professor. Not long after this appointment, Pincus claimed to have produced in vitro fertilization of rabbit eggs. In 1936, during Harvard's 300-year celebration of its founding, Pincus' work was lauded as one of the greatest scientific achievements in the history of the institution. In an astonishing about-face, Pincus, who was temporarily working again at Cambridge, was denied promotion to associate professor, effectively ending his employment at Harvard. There was, and still is, much speculation on the reason or reasons. Unfortunately, Pincus' work on in vitro fertilization of rabbit eggs coincided with the publication of Aldous Huxley's sensational and powerfully controversial novel, "Brave New World," wherein fetuses, conceived in vitro, were grown in laboratory bottles, each programmed to a set social stratum. As a result, Pincus became the focus of public hysteria over the possibility of his work being extrapolated to humans. In addition, there were undercurrents of anti-Semitism and professional jealousy, but perhaps the most damning indictment was that his experiment could not be duplicated. Indeed, later Chang was unable repeat Pincus' work. It should also be noted that promotion to full professorship at Harvard was far from guaranteed, particularly in one so young. Even so, Pincus' work was so outstanding that his prospects were unusually good.

Hoagland, now chairman of biology at Clark University, was deeply angry and offended at the treatment of his friend. In 1938, he offered Pincus a tenuously funded post as a visiting professor of zoology at Clark and privately raised the funds to support his appointment. These monies came from Nathaniel Lord Rothschild, who had worked at Cambridge with Pincus, and from a wealthy business friend of Hoagland's. After the attack on Pearl Harbor on 7th December, 1941, and with the onset of hostilities, Pincus and Hoagland did complementary research related to the ongoing war, Pincus working on hormonal responses to combat fatigue and Hoagland on nervous system responses. During this time Pincus and Hoagland communicated frequently, but with the end of the war their careers diverged, Hoagland becoming increasingly involved in administration and fund-raising.

By 1944, Hoagland and Pincus had become disenchanted with the situation at Clark University. They were at loggerheads with an overbearing administrator and caviled at having to teach prescribed courses to unenthusiastic students. There were also stressful faculty meetings characterized by bickering and petty jealousies. Together they launched a nonprofit corporation and formed the Worcester Foundation for Experimental Biology located at the little-known local hospital in Shrewsbury. At this time, it was difficult enough to raise funds for research in major universities, not to mention an obscure laboratory, but Hoagland secured some $25,000 for a building that was actually an old mansion, where, at first, the only workers were Pincus and Hoagland. It is widely reported that they employed themselves in janitorial and grounds keeping work to defray expenses. Nevertheless, within a short period of time, they were able to attract grants from the federal government, the National Cancer Research Center and crucially and prophetically from G.D. Searle[3], the pharmaceutical company that ultimately was the first to market the birth control pill. Altogether they raised $100,000 in the first year of operation. Through continuous research, Pincus, working with Chang, was able to show first that progesterone, given by injection, inhibited ovulation in mammals and later, that chemically altered progesterone was effective when given orally.

Progesterone, the elusive hormone that ultimately became the source of the contraceptive pill, did not spring suddenly into human

---

3   At the time, Searle was a small pharmaceutical company that provided hundreds of thousands of dollars for Pincus' unsuccessful research in the hope of biological conversion of serum into cortisone. His failure led to an angry confrontation with Searle's director of research, Albert Raymond, and Raymond's refusal of further funds but not the needed materials. It is to be recorded that Searle ultimately made huge profits from the sale of Enovid, the first, and for two years, the only available oral contraceptive.

ken like Minerva from the head of Zeus. Its discovery and chemical definition had a long history, from the suspicion of its presence to its identification, its biological extraction from animals, chemical definition, and finally its manufacture in bulk. The story of its discovery could be said to begin with the observation by a Dr. Baird of Edinburgh who noted in 1887 that pregnant women did not ovulate. Thus a woman, already pregnant, cannot become pregnant with a second fetus during her gestation. It was also a common observation among 19th-century German livestock handlers that infertile cows could be made fertile by crushing the ovaries. This was done manually per rectum. In fact, although pragmatically successful, the operator was unknowingly destroying residual ovarian cysts of pregnancy, or corpora lutei, whose output of progesterone inhibited fertility. While it is reported that the practice was widespread in animal husbandry throughout the latter part of 19th-century Europe, there is no known written record of the procedure.

In the early 1920s, Ludwig Haberlandt, professor of physiology at the University of Innsbruck, used ovarian and placental (afterbirth) extracts containing progesterone in both women and animals for regulation of fertility. He went so far as to market this extract under the name of Infecundin, but his early death in 1932 ended this endeavor. One would think that his discovery would have excited the widespread interest of other investigators, but this was in a different age in which the English-speaking world paid scant attention to European publications, not the least due to language and translation problems. However, progesterone, the active hormone responsible, was identified in the 1920s. It was not until several years later, in 1934, that the hormone was isolated and chemically defined contemporaneously by several separate investigators. In 1937 Dr.

A.W. Makepeace[4] showed that the hormone, given by subcutaneous injection, inhibited ovulation in rabbits. This work was aided by the convenient physiology of the female rabbit, which ovulates on coition. Makepeace's experiments were largely ignored by the scientific community, not least because progesterone was more expensive than gold. Moreover, as a potential contraceptive tool, it raised the question of acceptability. For example, what woman would submit to daily injections to prevent pregnancy even if progesterone were cheap and widely available? Moreover, even supposing a cheap progesterone, the price of daily injections would still be prohibitive in terms of syringes and medical costs. While significant, Makepeace's work was not quite revolutionary. In his own words he noted that many authors had produced evidence that the presence of a functional corpus luteum prevented ovulation in most mammalian species. What was significant was that he showed that progesterone was the active agent of the corpus luteum. This he did using varying doses of accurately measured progesterone chemically extracted from stigmasterol, found in the oils of certain plants such as soybeans, rape seed and calabar but also a variant extracted biologically from animals, specifically sows' ovaries. The latter was less precise in measurement because at the time, hormones were evaluated in terms of biological activity rather than in milligrams. In Makepeace's experiment, each product was effective no matter the dose. Because of this and other experimentation, Makepeace was able to conclude that the mechanism of action of progesterone was to inhibit the release of the pituitary hormone necessary for induction of ovulation. (It is interesting to note that after suppression of ovulation, Makepeace was able to induce ovulation in his rabbits by administering pituitary extract, the foundation of treatment of infertility some 20 or 30 years

4   1) American Journal of Physiology 119:512 1937

later.) Other investigators followed, showing a similar effect in rats (1939) and sheep (1948).

Of course, like any good researcher, Pincus was careful to review any published literature before embarking on his own experimentation. In 1951 he burdened an unenthusiastic Chang, hitherto focused on fertilization, with inquiring into the effect of progesterone, now, thanks to the work of Russell Marker, cheaper and more readily available, on rabbit ovulation. Despite the necessary and expensive sacrifice of his rabbit subjects in order to determine the success of progesterone administration, as time went by, Chang became increasingly interested in the results. In a paper published in 1953 (Acta Phys. Latinoam), he and Pincus showed that progesterone administered subcutaneously was not only completely effective in inhibiting ovulation in rabbits, but that this was dose-related and related also to the time of administration, for example low doses and late administration following coitus were shown to be incompletely effective. Chang and Pincus in their paper also noted the effect of other similar hormones, finding them less effective than progesterone. Of even more interest, longstanding inhibition of ovulation in the rabbit could be accomplished by subcutaneous implantation of pellets containing progesterone.

It was relatively easy to perform such experiments on rabbits by virtue of their unique ovulatory response to coitus. Pincus, in a paper published in 1956 (Acta endocrinology supplementum XXVIII), showed that this was also true in rats. In the same paper written by Pincus as sole author, but quoting gynecologist John Rock, he describes the suppressive effect of oral progesterone in human females. Effective in a high proportion of women, and with increasing effectiveness from month to month, nevertheless, the regime was clearly insufficiently reliable as an effective contraceptive measure.

Further experimentation on rabbits described in the same paper using a variety of artificial progesterones, or progestins, showed two progestins to be effective by mouth. One of these was Frank Colton's norethynodrel, now patented by the Searle company, later absorbed by Pfizer. The other, of which more later, was norethindrone, produced by an obscure laboratory in Mexico named Syntex. Pincus, again in the same paper, showed that norethynodrel by mouth effectively suppressed ovulation in a small series of four women. At the conclusion of his paper, he acknowledged the contributions of Rock and his colleagues at the Free Hospital for Women.

Now, it was apparent that these progestins could, after oral administration, inhibit ovulation but were they safe or could they produce unacceptable side effects?

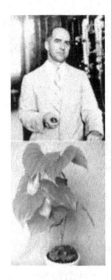

CHAPTER FIVE

The Chemists
Russell Marker
Dioscorea Mexicana

We have reviewed the history of progesterone from the time of recognition of the biological action of the corpus luteum to the identification of its active factor progesterone and thereafter to the identification of the chemical configuration of progesterone itself in 1934. Exciting as these discoveries were, biological experimentation was inhibited by the sheer cost of the hormone, which in the 1940s was, at $8 per gram, more expensive than gold. At that time, progesterone was extracted either from sows' ovaries, an expensive and tedious process, or by cumbersome chemical manipulation of cholesterol and bile acids. Into the picture now comes Russell Marker, an enigmatic, elusive and controversial character who nevertheless was a brilliant research chemist. Nobody has written a definitive biography of this fascinating individual, although an aura of legend has grown up around his pursuits, pursuits that he often carried out alone and secretively. However, he did leave some brief autobiographical notes. In addition, two extensive interviews were conducted by Bernard Asbell in 1992 when Marker was then 89 and by Jeffrey Sturchio in April of 1987. Aside from these, we are dependent on his brief and casual biographical notes dated May 1969 and some side comments by other authors intent on the pursuit of alternative avenues of enquiry. What is well established is that he was born on 12th March, 1902, in a one-room log cabin on a 40-acre farm located about seven miles east of Hagerstown, Maryland, where his father worked as a sharecropper. Farming had been a family occupation since Marker's great-great-grandfather George Marker emigrated from northern Germany.

Russell Marker attended the local grade school in Maugansville, where upon completion of eighth grade, students were permitted to write the examinations given to high school students at the end of ninth grade and, if a pass was obtained, the student could be admitted directly to 10th grade. In this, Marker was successful. To get to high school, he had to walk two miles to a train station, take the train, then walk one mile to the school. To catch the 07:15 a.m. train, Marker had to be on his way by 6:30. His high school education was quite basic and took the form of commercial courses only. He was given no education in physics, chemistry or botany. Following Marker's graduation from Hagerstown High School in 1919, his father had wanted him to settle down on the family farm but, in defiance of his father's wishes and with an abhorrence of farm work, he applied and was accepted at the University of Maryland.

Admission to the University of Maryland was facilitated in part by a dearth of applicants in the year 1919 after the 1918 end of World War I. A sympathetic registrar gave him provisional admission conditional upon completion of classes in English and mathematics at summer school, which Marker undertook, achieving good grades. With no notion of what was involved, he chose chemical engineering as his major without even the most basic knowledge of laboratory materials unable as he was to recognize something as simple as a test tube. He changed after the first year to regular chemistry. Despite this, by the third and fourth years his grades were largely A's with a scattering of B's.

At the end of his sophomore year in the university's School of Chemistry, Marker became attracted to the discipline of organic chemistry. He decided to take classes in this field in his junior year. Forewarned by the professor of organic chemistry that he was about to recommend a certain textbook by Harris, and having been advised of the difficulty of the course, Marker purchased the book in advance of classes. During the summer recess he covered its contents entirely, working out the problems at the end of each chapter. During that junior year, Marker found organic chemistry to be the easiest and most interesting of his chemical courses. It is significant that, in particular, the laboratory work drew his greatest attention. He graduated with a B.S. in chemistry in 1923. His career decision was prophetic of Marker's single-mindedness and independence, for in life he would pursue courses of action based on his intellectual interests to the exclusion of others, whether financial or social. After graduation, unable to secure the only fellowship available in organic chemistry, he was offered one in physical chemistry enabling him to graduate with an M.S. in 1924.

Upon completion of his M.S. and under the aegis of noted chemist Morris Kharasch, who offered him a fellowship in organic chemistry at $1,000 per year, he began doctoral studies, finishing these with a dissertation on organic mercurials. However, his dissertation was not published until 1928, when, with the assistance of Kharasch, it was accepted by the Journal of the American Chemical Society. But Marker never achieved doctoral status, which in the words of Djerassi (see below) constituted the "union card" of the academic chemist. Notwithstanding that Marker had completed all the work required for his thesis, Kharasch told him that, to be eligible for his doctorate, he would be required to take additional mandatory courses in physical chemistry and pass the examinations. Deeming such studies duplicative and redundant, and against the advice of Kharasch, he left the university in June of 1925 never to achieve his doctorate. Kharasch made dire predictions that his subsequent career would consist of performing prosaic and commonplace chemistry such as urinalysis. Kharasch, by the way, was no mean chemist himself. Among his successes in the course of a brilliant career was the preparation and patenting of the mercurial compound thimerosal, which, until recently, was widely used as a preservative in vaccines. In this he was assisted by Marker. Kharasch also produced a compound called mercurochrome. This product, under the trade name of Merthiolate, was widely used as an antiseptic in operating rooms in the '50s and beyond. (This author has fond memories of its peculiarly translucent reddish pink color and of its distinctive, pungent but not unpleasant odor.)

Kharasch's predictions were not entirely amiss. Marker indeed, found it difficult to secure remunerative employment. He took a position at the Naval Powder Factory at Indian Head, Md., to tide himself over until he could find something better. Having married Mildred Collins in 1926, Marker was eager to take the position that paid $2,000 per year. After five months at the Powder Factory, he was offered a job at the Ethyl Corporation in Yonkers at $2,600 per year starting on 1st February, 1926. During his time there, he was to meet Frank Whitmore, later to become his employer at Pennsylvania State University. The Ethyl Corporation had been recently formed as a subdivision of General Motors. Automobile engines were then troubled by "knocking," a vibration noted on acceleration or going uphill. Tetra Ethyl lead was then used in gasoline as an anti-knock agent. It was thought that Marker, having some familiarity with metallic organic compounds, would be useful in exploring alternative anti knock agents. He met with Dr. Graham Edgar, project head, in an old abandoned garage in Yonkers that the company had rented to convert into their first laboratory. However, he was told not to report for work for two months in order to allow time for installation of laboratory benches and equipment. When he did start work on 1st February, 1926, he found that neither glassware nor chemicals were available. While awaiting this correction, Marker nosed around the gasoline testing laboratory. Noting that the mixed hydrocarbons used for engine testing had a variable boiling point, he exchanged them for a pure hydrocarbon that had a definitive boiling point. This was n-heptane (seven carbon chain), which, alas, caused extreme knocking. Marker concluded that odd-numbered hydrocarbons were more likely to do this, so he decided to make an octane (8 carbon chain). Tertiary butyl alcohol was readily available and by chemical manipulation of this raw material, he was able to produce the octane 2,2,4-trimethylpentene and reduce this to 2,2,4 tri methyl pentane. Use of this product eliminated knocking. It was further found that a mixture of 80% octane with 20% heptane met the current standards for a gasoline with anti-knock properties. Thus did Marker establish the octane number still today a standard for the quality of gasoline. This activity alone would have established Marker as a chemist of note. Going further into this field, he found that gasoline consisting solely of octanes still had bad knocking problems. He resolved this problem by "branching" the octanes.[5]

The oil-refining companies immediately took advantage of his findings to change their practices to produce the maximum number of branched chain hydrocarbons and raise the octane number. It was toward the end of his time at Ethyl that Frank Whitmore dropped by for a half-day expressing interest in Marker's work. At the end of the day, he asked Marker to look him up should he ever want a job at Penn State, where Whitmore eventually became dean.

After two years, and despite a salary increase to $3,300 per year, bored with hydrocarbons at Ethyl, Marker went to work in February of 1928 at the renowned Rockefeller Institute for Medical Research, later to become the Rockefeller University. Founded in 1901, the institute had as its only goal the furthering of biomedical research. He was assigned to work under Phoebus A. Levene (1869-1940), head of the chemistry department. Levene was a noted investigator responsible for chemically defining nucleotides, the building blocks of DNA. He had approached Marker in August of 1927, inviting him to an informal meeting at his apartment where, during the interview, he presented Marker with a complex chemical problem based on the Walden Inversion, for which Marker immediately foresaw the solution. On the following day at lunch with Levene and Dr. Simon Flexner[6], the director of the Rockefeller Institute, he was offered a

---

5   The simplest hydrocarbons (alkanes) are formed from carbon atoms linked in linear fashion (C-C-C-C-C-_C etc.), but with chemical manipulation these can be "branched".   C-C-C-C-C
$$\text{C-C-C-C-C} \atop | \atop \text{C}$$

6   Dr. Simon Flexner was a prominent pathologist after whom Shigella Flexner, the bacterium responsible for a severe form of dysentery, was named. His younger brother, Abraham, a noted educator, was the author of the famous 1910 Flexner Report responsible for review and reform of medical education in the United States.

salary of $4,000 per year equal to an offer that had recently been made to him by an industrial company, but in addition, included two months of annual vacation. He was allowed to give Ethyl sixth months' notice, so that he did not start work at the institute until 1st February of 1928. It was characteristic of Marker's intellectual curiosity that he worked throughout the two months of his summer vacation completing his research on the problems of the so-called Walden Inversion.

While spending his six years at the Rockefeller Institute, Marker, with Levene, published more than 25 papers. It was during this time that his attention was drawn to steroid research. Dr. Walter Jacobs, who worked in the laboratory adjacent to Marker, had done some pioneer work on steroids, the basis of many biological hormones such as testosterone, estrogen, progesterone and cortisone, but had also worked on certain plant steroids known as sapogenins. However, the plant steroids had a chemical side chain, which Jacobs, along with several other German scientists, had concluded was impossible to remove in order to produce a pure hormone. Nevertheless, Marker saw the need for production of these steroid hormones at much lower cost. In the spring of 1935, he requested a change in his work to accommodate his interest. Levene declined his proposals, so Marker told Levene that he intended to leave if not permitted to do so. The director of the institute, Dr. Flexner was not only irked but also perplexed that Marker would even consider leaving such a prestigious and well-paid position at the renowned institute. After an angry confrontation with Flexner, while Marker was precipitously packing to leave, Levene came to Marker's office and persuaded him to stay until he could take up a contract with Penn State, so that Marker remained at the institute until September, completing as far as possible, his assigned research, working conscientiously throughout his two months of summer vacation. Later he compiled these results for publication while serving his first three months at Penn State. This change was another example of Marker's refusal to be bound by the strictures of secure employment.

As we have already noted, while working at Ethyl, Marker had met Dr. Frank Whitmore, now the dean of chemistry at Penn State. Whitmore had long ago invited him to visit him should he ever have thoughts of changing employment. So, with the offer of a fellowship, Marker began work at Penn State on 1st September in a post that was funded by research grants from the pharmaceutical company Parke-Davis. The move was doubly astonishing, for at the Rockefeller Institute, he had had the comfortable salary of $4,400 per annum including two months' vacation, whereas the fellowship at Penn State paid only $1,800. When you also take into account that this was in 1935 at the bottom of the depression with a scarcity of jobs of any kind, one gathers either a profound respect for Marker's lack of interest in pecuniary gain or perhaps reservations regarding his fiscal acumen. More likely it was a reflection of his intellectual curiosity, a curiosity that discounted the distractions of monetary compensation, a pattern repeated throughout his career

Upon arrival at Penn State, he was faced with primitive laboratory conditions and little help. Progesterone had already been produced in small amounts from cholesterol in a laborious and expensive process known as degradation, wherein much of the chemical structure of cholesterol was split off, leaving the hormone. Finding a kilogram of cholesterol in a storage area, Marker, while awaiting the arrival of more sophisticated apparatus, occupied his time by repeating the degradation process described by Swiss and German chemists suffi-ciently to realize that such would never produce progesterone in large amounts. His research progressed with the isolation of the steroid pregnanediol from the urine of pregnant cows and mares. (Pregnanediol is a steroid closely allied chemically to progesterone and is a metabolite of that hormone. Today its detection in urine may be used as confirmation of ovulation. Pregnant animals, including humans, excrete pregnanediol in large amounts.) From this steroid, Marker was able to extract a significant amount of progesterone, in fact more than had ever been produced before in one lot. At the then-current price, adjusted for inflation, of $1,000 per gram, his 35-gram extract was worth $35,000. (Gold in the '30s sold for about $11 per gram.) These 35 grams were remitted and sold to Parke-Davis, offsetting the costs of Marker's research fellowship by a considerable margin. Progesterone was at that time much in demand by experimental physiologists for the investigation and treatment of menstrual disorders, problem pregnancies and even some forms of gynecologic cancer, but was too expensive for casual use. However gynecological interest was merely a side issue to the potential of converting progesterone into cortisone, an adrenal gland hormone useful as an anti-inflammatory agent, particularly in the treatment of rheumatoid arthritis, a crippling illness without any cure. Cortisone produces the most remarkable remissions of the disease and was widely utilized until it became apparent that long-term use caused severe complications.

Marker, as we have noted, through his association with Jacobs at the Rockefeller Institute had acquired some familiarity with sapogenins, a collective name for a group of similar botanical chemicals. Chemically they have a nuclear ring similar to pregnanediol, which Marker knew could easily be converted to progesterone. However, the sapogenins have a chemical side chain, which at that time was assumed by Jacobs to be inert and impossible to remove. This chemical side chain was defined by two German chemists Tschesche and Hagedorn whose work was repeated by American chemists Louis F. Feiser[7] and Jacobson of Harvard on the side chain of sarsasapogenin, which seemed to confirm "beyond any doubt" the inertia of the side chain. But on careful review of their publications, Marker concluded that they were wrong. Repeating their work he correctly defined the nature of the side chain effectively removing it by boiling the substrate under pressure overnight with acetic anhydride leaving him with the progesterone-like substance, pregneneolone acetate, which he easily reduced to pregnanedione, a substance closely related to progesterone and an excellent substrate for conversion to the hormone. This description of his work is trite and abbreviated and does not take account of the many hours and multiple laboratory experiments involved. Even at the conclusion, seeking confirmation, Marker had to send the end product to New York for verification.

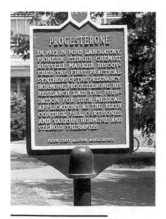

This process supplemented the supply of progesterone to Parke-Davis, whose company president, Dr. Alexander Lescohier, was duly impressed. In addition, it was later found that pregneneolone could be converted into a variety of male hormones, including testosterone. Marker's remarkable accomplishment was a watershed in steroid chemistry and was

7   Louis F. Fieser was a towering, energetic, figure in the field of organic chemistry noted for his work not only on steroids, but on Vitamin K, blood clotting factors, and later on napalm. He was a professor at Harvard who, in the course of his career, published many of the standard textbooks used by chemists. It is small wonder that he looked askance at the work of a maverick investigator like Marker who worked at a relatively obscure institution and didn't even have a doctorate. In his interview by Sturchio, Marker recalls that he was invited to dinner by Feiser and his wife, but when Feiser learned earlier in the day of Marker's degradation process, he became quiet angry, did not show for the scheduled dinner, and left his wife to dine alone with Marker.

quickly published in a three-paragraph entry in the Journal of the American Chemistry Society to the great irritation of Louis Feiser who, despite the accuracy of the work, remained a recalcitrant skeptic. A plaque outside the Pond building at Penn State records Marker's historical work as the Marker Degradation (see photo). But for Marker, the barrier to greater production was not the chemical process, but a richer source of sapogenins. Until this time he had used the root of the sasparilla plant collected in limited quantities from Mexico. Moreover, effective as his process was, it was still an expensive method of production.

Meantime, upon completion of his first year at Penn State, he was given a staff appointment at a salary of $2,400 so that he now used his $1,800 fellowship money to buy chemicals and for excursions in the pursuit of substitute botanicals for sasparilla. The fellowship remuneration from Parke-Davis was later increased to $10,000, but as Marker observed, his earlier production of 35 grams of progesterone at $1,000 per gram more than offset the cost of his fellowship from Parke-Davis. Marker continued working at Penn State until 1943, by which time he held a full professorship at $4,000 per year, but during the previous four years he occupied much of his time in the search for better botanical sources of sapogenins both in the United States and Mexico. At every meeting of chemists he attended he solicited sources of sapogenins so that his laboratory soon became redolent of the fragrances or sometimes the noxious odors of those botanicals. From one particular sapogenin that became known as diogenin, Marker could easily extract progesterone.

During a visit to the home of one of the botanists assisting in the collection of plants in Texas for the purpose of extracting sapogenins, significantly, one Japanese chemist sent him a specimen of a plant group known as dioscorea. Marker's attention was drawn to the picture of a large dioscorea that grew in Mexico and developed a root size of 100 kilograms. This so called cabeza de negro was named for the similarity of its surface protrusions which resembled the crinkled hair of a negro. The exact geographical location of the so called cabeza de negro plant in the southern area of Mexico was unknown. The state of Vera Cruz was given, so Marker, funded by a reluctant and skeptical Whitmore, went first to Mexico City in November of 1941 in search of the plant.

The American Embassy in Mexico City was unhelpful, telling Marker that he would have to have a permit from the Mexican government for plant collection and that this would be difficult because of the pro-German stance of the Mexican government during World War II, which had begun on September of 1939. In November 1941, the Japanese attack on Pearl Harbor was now only a month away. In addition, he was asked to have typhoid immunization prior to going to the site of his investigations because of the prevalence there of that disease. Marker returned to the U.S. empty-handed.

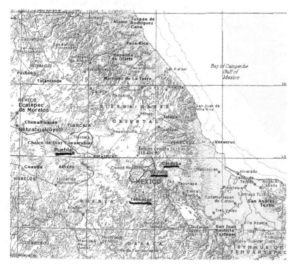

Marker persisted. He went back to Mexico in January of 1942 and later gave an account of his adventures in search of the elusive inedible yam cabeza de negro. Circumventing the license requirement, he described how the American Embassy suggested that he enlist the services of a Mexican botanist, who apparently was also without a permit for plant collection, but would accompany him to the state of Vera Cruz, the presumed but uncertain, location of the recondite cabeza de negro, at a location almost 200 miles southeast of Mexico City. Toward this purpose, Marker rented a truck with a driver, but the botanist, who spoke no English, arrived at his hotel in a car accompanied by an interpreter. The transportation issue was further complicated by the additional accompaniment of the botanist's girlfriend and her mother acting as a chaperone! The botanist insisted that he would not go unless he had these traveling companions with him. Expecting no more than a three-day trip, Marker reluctantly agreed. However, on the first day they traveled a mere 80 miles to the southeast, reaching Puebla, where they stayed overnight. On the second day the travelling distance was even shorter, reaching Tehuacan[8], where the botanist insisted on staying two nights. Worse, after the two-night stay the botanist told Marker that there was local resistance to further travel because Marker was American. On the return to Mexico City the vehicle broke down near Puebla. Thus, Marker arrived back in Mexico City after a week of travel without any of the sought-after plants. Reporting these vicissitudes to the American embassy, Marker was advised to forget about his plans in this quixotic search for an elusive yam. Instead, on the Monday evening of his return, he took the bus back to Puebla, arriving there after midnight. The following morning he took a second, rickety bus to Orizaba. "It had pigs in the bottom and the woman in the seat beside me had some chickens with her," he told Sturchio. From Orizaba he took yet another bus trip to Cordoba. The botany text had described the plant's location on the banks of a stream that ran through a ravine bridged by the road between Orizaba and Cordoba. Recognizing the stream from the botanical description, he exited the bus. He was successful in locating a nearby small country store owned by an Indian who spoke no English. Somehow, Marker got him to understand his interest in

---

8   A curious stopping point. The city is located quite far to the south of Marker's proposed destination. See map.

cabeza de negro and the next morning the Indian, Alberto Moreno, had secured for him two plants, each about 25 years old and weighing 50 pounds. Marker placed them in bags and loaded them on to the roof of the bus returning to Orizaba. Upon arriving in Orizaba he found that both bags were missing. Miraculously overcoming the language barrier with a local policeman, the production of a $10 bill resulted in one of the bags being recovered. Lacking a second $10, Marker had to be satisfied with the exchange although one is left to wonder to what use the thief would put this inedible plant. The remaining retrieved plant never left Marker's sight until he arrived back in Pennsylvania, where he personally chopped it up, dried it, and extracted a sapogenin from half of the root. He took the remaining half to Parke-Davis in Detroit. He proposed on-site extraction in Mexico to Dr. Alexander Lescohier, the president of Parke Davis, who was resistant to Marker's suggestion even although Parke-Davis owned a building in Mexico City. A small part of the building could easily have been adapted to Marker's purpose. Incredibly, Marker could not interest Parke-Davis in commercializing this process. It was the opinion of the president that bull's urine was an adequate source of progesterone production and indeed, given the then-prevalent view of Mexico as a backward country, Lescohier probably felt quite justified in his stance. In fact, during an earlier visit to Mexico, Lescohier had become seriously ill with appendicitis and was quite contemptuous of the quality of the medical care provided him. Marker was further turned down by several other pharmaceutical companies, including Merck, Ciba and Schering-Plough, partly because they knew of the rejection by Parke-Davis, partly because they suspected, incorrectly, that Parke Davis had secured a patent on the degradation process. Convinced that the only way in which hormones could be made in Mexico was if he did it himself, in October 1942 Marker withdrew half of his limited savings account and returned to Mexico, where he contacted Alberto Moreno. The latter soon secured for him the enormous amount of 10 tons of cabeza de negro. Moreno, at Marker's direction and using only machetes, chopped up the material into small amounts "like potato chips" that were then sun-dried, reducing the weight in the process to two tons. This material he took to Mexico City, where he found someone with a crude extractor. The dried material was extracted with alcohol and Marker transported the resultant syrup to New York where, with the promise of sharing one third of the progesterone product, he entered into an arrangement with a friend, Norman Applezweig, for the free use of his laboratory and staff. (Applezweig was already a noted biochemist in his own right and later went on to found the pharmaceutical company Progenics.)

The syrup was refined to produce the largest amount of progesterone known at that time — three kilograms, almost one kilogram more than Marker had anticipated — at a recorded value of $240,000, or $80 per gram. In return for the use of his lab, he donated one kilogram to Applezweig. It is not clear from the records what Marker did with the remaining two kilograms, but it seemed to play a part in his later negotiations with the man who would become his business partner, Emeric Somlo.

In his much-later interview with Carl Djerassi (Oct. 1979), Marker told him how he established a laboratory in Mexico City for the commercial production of progesterone. He had gone back to Mexico during 1943 and under great difficulty had produced three kilograms of progesterone, two of which went to Somlo's Laboratorios Hormonos and one to a pharmaceutical distributor in the U.S. who later became his partner in a company called Botanica-Mex.

Seeking a laboratory in Mexico City for continuing production, Marker simply went to the telephone directory and looked up "Laboratorios" in the business pages. Stumbling on Laboratorios Hormonos, he took a taxi to its location and met with the scientific director, Federico Lehmann, who, with vague memories of having seen Marker's name in scientific publications, quickly confirmed this when he retrieved a copy of the Journal of the American Chemistry Society.

Lehmann, an employee with a medical degree and a Ph.D., contacted the owner of the laboratory, Somlo, who was then in New York, asking him to come immediately to Mexico City. Somlo, a small businessman and former lawyer from Hungary who had assumed the spurious title of Doctor, arrived within a day or two, having learned that Marker had produced a small amount of progesterone as proof of his work. Marker describes in his biographical notes how a rough contract was drawn up between him and Laboratorios Hormonos pending his availability and release from his obligations at Penn State. This relatively obscure occurrence was the foundation of the famous pharmaceutical company called Syntex. In his interview with Djerassi much later in October 1979, Marker stated that neither Somlo nor Lehmann knew that he had made some progesterone in the U.S. Marker returned to the U.S. for several months to finish up his research at Penn State.

In September of 1943 Marker submitted his resignation from the faculty at the School of Chemistry at Penn State College effective 1st December, which was ultimately accepted after he refused the counter offer of the position of assistant dean. At an undefined time in 1943, but presumably in the fall, Marker, back in Mexico City but about to return to the States, mentioned to a greatly surprised Lehmann that he had made several kilos of progesterone in the U.S. Not only that, but he further added that he still had this in his possession. Back in the States he received a phone call from Somlo who, on learning that Marker still had progesterone in his possession, invited him to a dinner meeting at the Waldorf Astoria in Marker's words, to "butter him up." Marker took two kilograms of his progesterone to Chemical Specialties, a small company Somlo owned in New York, where its nature was confirmed and for which he was given a receipt. Somlo evaluated the progesterone at a price of $80 per gram ($160,000). He proposed a business contract whereby Marker, Somlo and Lehmann would form a stock company for further production of the hormone in Mexico City. The significant clauses of the contract were that the company would be floated with a capital of 500,000 pesos, or about $100,000. Somlo would hold a controlling interest of 52%, while Marker's interest would be 40% ($40,000), to be funded by the sale of his two kilograms of progesterone ($160,000), with the remaining 8% held by Lehmann. The balance of Marker's $120,000 contribution was to go to the company profits, shared on the basis of percentage ownership, as would all subsequent income after deductions for overhead. The company, at Marker's suggestion, was named Syntex as an indication of its location in Mexico.

However, after a year in which Marker was paid sporadically such as when he needed money for his hotel bills or to travel home to his wife and family in the U.S., he requested his share of the profits from Somlo. Although Marker had produced 30 kilograms of progesterone, Somlo declared that there were no profits and refused to disclose the accounts to Marker, alleging that he would be unable to understand them given his lack of accounting experience complicated by the fact that they were compiled in Spanish. No one has ever formally accused Somlo of exploiting Marker, but if we assume the market value of progesterone to be $25 per gram, the lower of Marker's estimated value during that year of production, then the gross income for the year would have been $750,000 (30,000 x $25). Lehman's and Somlo's shares of the gross would then have totaled $450,000 (52%+8%=60%) leaving a balance of $300,000, surely enough to pay for Marker's initial investment of $40,000, reimburse him $140,000 in profit, and still leave $120,000 for his share of overhead. ($750,000 x 40%). Of course, we can only guess at overhead costs. Nor can we be sure that the exact price of progesterone was $25 per gram. We leave readers to draw their own conclusions but Marker left the company immediately in May of 1945.[9]

---

9   Much later, at a chemical meeting in 1991, Pedro Lehman a chemist and son of Federico Lehmann, gave a screen projection that showed that Marker had been paid $17,500 in 1943 or '44, but whether as salary or expenses was not clarified. Even so, it would seem to represent only a small proportion of Marker's contribution.

In a curious but portentous side issue, Marker had agreed with Parke-Davis to sign patent applications no later than 15th December, 1943, conditional upon completion of a formal agreement. This did not occur, but the patent attorney came to meet with Marker in Mexico City in April of 1944, bringing with him more than 30 patent applications for signature, which Marker refused to sign. The director of research at Parke-Davis, a good friend of Marker's, was subsequently expedited to Mexico City to persuade Marker into signing. He was conducted to Marker's relatively primitive laboratory where he had for help some four ill-educated young Mexican women who produced from Marker's supplies, a bottle with two kilograms of the precious progesterone that these uneducated girls had made under Marker's direction. The director called Detroit and was told to offer Marker liberal royalties would he but sign the patent agreements. Once more Marker refused. It was his position that a patent would prevent worldwide competition in progesterone production, thus preventing an appropriate reduction in price!

Who can guess at Marker's reason? Was he truly motivated by altruistic concerns that the pharmaceutical industry should not profit from his discovery at the expense of consumers, or was this another example of his cantankerous irascibility?

After his disagreement with Somlo and departure from Syntex, taking with him his former staff of four Mexican girls, in May of 1945 Marker founded his own company, Botanica-Mex in Texcoco, finding an even better source of diosgenin in another dioscorea, the barbasco plant. In fact, barbasco proved to be a source four times as great as the cabeza de negro. There is much suspicion of the actions of his competition. His native collector of barbasco was shot dead, and one of his two night watchmen was shot through the leg. In Texcoco, he continued to produce progesterone to a total of about 30 kilograms, or the same amount that he had produced at Syntex, until March of 1946, when production was moved to Mexico City under the auspices of the Hungarian pharmaceutical company, Gideon Richter. Gideon Richter in turn formed a subsidiary company called Hormosynth, later changed to Diosynth. Meantime Botanica-Mex was liquidated. It is to be noted at this point that Marker, never having patented his extraction process in Mexico, had thus cleared the way for Syntex to produce progesterone independently. However, only Marker knew the process. Upon leaving Syntex, and not for the first time in his career, he had removed the labels from his reagents, an act considered in research chemistry to be so highly reprehensible as to border on delinquency. Syntex meantime hired Dr. George Rosenkranz as his replacement.

Compare the structure with norethindrone and norethynodrel for similarity.

Norethynodrel

Norethindrone

The only difference between the steroids norethindrone and norethynodrel is the location of the double bond in the first A six carbon ring.

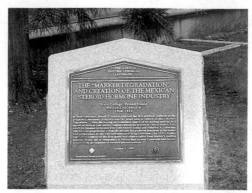

The text reads: The "Marker Degradation" and
the creation of the Mexican Steroid industry.
State College, Pennsylvania
Mexico City, Mexico

In Pond Laboratory, Russell Marker achieved the first practical synthesis of the pregnancy hormone, progesterone, by what is now known as the "Marker Degradation." After discovering an economical source of the starting material in a species of Mexican yam, Marker commercialized his process in 1944 at Syntex S.A., which he founded in Mexico City with Emeric Somlo and Federico A. Lehman. The low-cost progesterone eventually became the preferred precursor in the industrial preparation of the anti-inflammatory drug cortisone. In 1951, Syntex researchers synthesized the first useful oral contraceptive from Marker's starting material. Syntex and its competitors in Mexico thus became a powerful international force in the development of steroidal pharmaceuticals.

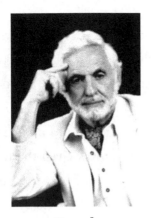

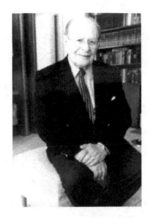

Carl Djerassi

George Rosenkranz

George Rosenkranz was a Hungarian Jewish fugitive from the Europe of World War II. He had earned his doctorate in technical sciences in 1940 at the prestigious Swiss Federal Institute of Technology in Zurich under the tutelage of Leopold Ruzicka, who was later to become a Nobel Laureate. Ruzicka was yet another brilliant investigator of steroids who became something of a mentor to Rosenkranz but also a protector of him and his several Jewish colleagues. Despite Swiss neutrality, Rosenkranz and his fellow Jewish chemists were subjected to the disapprobation of their ethnicity so acute in neighboring Nazi Germany that several of them determined to leave Switzerland. Most chose to emigrate to the United States, but Rosenkranz accepted an offer as chairman of organic chemistry in Quito, Ecuador. This aspiration was frustrated when, while he was en route, the Japanese attacked Pearl Harbor. Stuck in Havana, he was saved by the intervention of Cuban President Fulgencio Batista, who issued a decree granting residency status to all refugees. Rosenkranz took a post with the largest pharmaceutical company on the island, ultimately becoming its director of research. Familiar with the work of Marker, Rosenkranz tinkered with some sasparilla and was able to extract a small amount of progesterone. Word of this reached the ears of Somlo and Lehmann who, desperate to restart the lucrative production of progesterone, invited Rosenkranz to Mexico City for a job interview. This took place on 6th August, 1945, a date incidentally unique in history for the destruction of Hiroshima by the atomic bomb. As a test of his abilities, he was given the task of the last chemical step in laboratory production of progesterone. Hardly a challenging proposition for Rosenkranz, he quickly and expeditiously accomplished this to the astonishment of Somlo and Lehmann, who immediately offered him a job. Any hesitation by Rosenkranz was based on the knowledge that he would first have to determine the nature of the unlabeled reagents used by Marker, no simple task, but his work in Cuba had been even less attractive, so that he decided to accept. As a measure of his confidence, in short order, he telephoned his girlfriend in Havana and proposed marriage, a union that persists to this day. In his daydreams, he pictured Syntex as becoming a major source of pharmaceuticals, but never in the most wild of these dreams did he foresee the astonishing success that was to come. Within two months he had solved the riddle of Marker's reagents and had started the production of progesterone. Within two years he had established mass production. By the late 1940s, Syntex was the major bulk supplier of progesterone to the world's foremost pharmaceutical companies

The steroid progesterone, at that time, was of little inherent interest. Rather it was seen as a potential substrate for the production of cortisone. In 1946 investigators at Merck had been successful in manufacturing a small amount of cortisone from animal sources by a tedious and expensive process. A larger amount was produced at the Mayo Clinic by a separate and more efficient method. What was of high importance was the revelation that cortisone had a dramatic effect on rheumatoid arthritis. The Mayo clinic made a movie of patients, hitherto bedridden with the disease, dancing on the floor after a single day of treatment! In addition, it was a favored precursor of the male hormone testosterone.

Progesterone had now become cheap. The fiscal roadblock to further biological experimentation had been removed. This was the significance of Marker's work. Doctors and biologists were now able to explore the therapeutic effects of the hormone while chemists had a cheap raw material for further manipulation of the progesterone molecule into cortisone. Indeed, in a short autobiographical note, Marker professed personal satisfaction in having found the source for production of abundant supplies of steroidal hormones, at low prices and without patents or royalties, thus opening the door to rapid expansion of steroids in the treatment of disease and in particular, the development of the oral contraceptive pill.

Carl Djerassi

The career of Carl Djerassi is more easily defined thanks to his engaging autobiographical work, "This Man's Pill." Even making allowances for the self-laudatory stance natural to any autobiography, he gives a fascinating and well-documented account of further steroidal developments leading to the contraceptive pill. Using the metaphor of conception, embryo implantation, fetal development and finally the birth of the pill, he downgrades Marker's contribution as that of a mere maternal grand uncle. However, while progesterone had long been chemically identified and artificially produced in steroid laboratories, it was Marker's genius to seek and find an alternative botanical resource of the hormone and to devise a means of mass production rendering this raw material available for chemical manipulation and medical experimentation. Even Djerassi acknowledges that, at one time, he recommended Marker for a Nobel Prize and that had it not been for Marker, there would have been no Syntex, which, at the time of his absorption into the company in the spring of 1949, was on the threshold of becoming a major pharmaceutical company.

In that particular spring, Djerassi, never having heard of Syntex, out of the blue received from the company an offer of employment. Almost as an article of faith, he responded to this offer from what was then an obscure company in a poor and backward third-world country. Contemporary Mexico was not then noted for steroidal research or indeed for much else in the way of scientific endeavor. However, being of an adventurous nature, combined with an offer of an all-expenses-paid trip to a tropical paradise, the recently married 22 year old accepted.

Djerassi was yet another Jewish immigrant from Europe. Born on 29th October, 1923, to a Bulgarian father and an Austrian mother, each a physician, he was raised in Vienna before coming to the U.S. Lacking even a high school diploma, he inveigled himself into acceptance at the Newark Junior College in pre-med. Hardly knowing a test tube from a Bunsen burner, he fell under the influence of a "superb" teacher of chemistry, Nathan Washton, and switched to that field. Moving eventually to Kenyon College in Ohio, he quickly graduated from there in 1942 with a B.A. in organic chemistry. Within a relatively short time, he achieved his doctorate from the University of Wisconsin in 1945 and went to work for CIBA pharmaceutical company in New Jersey, where he was allowed to spend 20% of his time in independent research. This led him to publish a fair amount of scientific literature. He aspired to enter the academic world of chemistry, not impossible, but no easy feat for an employee of a commercial laboratory.

He had been working for four years at CIBA at the time of the offer from Syntex, which he regarded as ludicrous. The obscure company was located in what he describes as "the professional backwater of Mexico." Despite his ingrained contempt, he was greatly impressed upon meeting with the 30-year-old Rosenkranz, if not by his primitive laboratory. Djerassi took up work in Mexico City in the late autumn of 1949 as assistant director of research. With the advent of cortisone and the later award in 1950 of a Nobel Prize to its discoverers, steroid chemistry was then a hot topic, so that this was the line of work that had engaged the attention of the 25-year-old Djerassi. Using the same yam substrate that Marker had used for progesterone, the two young researchers electrified the world in 1951 with a much-simplified and cheaper method for production of cortisone. This was published in the Journal of the American Chemical Society issue of August 1951. Impressive as such a finding was, almost immediately the Upjohn Company in Kalamazoo, Mich., announced an even simpler one-step process in the production of cortisone, ironically using progesterone as a substrate. Upjohn had ordered it in enormous bulk from Syntex, the only company that could meet the order for the huge amount, 10 tons, that it had requested. As reported by Djerassi, the entire world production at that time was less than one-hundredth of that amount. What Upjohn achieved was not by chemistry, but rather by the novel technique of bacteriological conversion of the progesterone substrate. However, if nothing else, the ability of Syntex to meet the huge request of Upjohn put its laboratory on the world map.

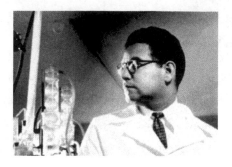

Luis Miramontes

Djerassi and Rosenkranz now turned their attention to manipulation of the progesterone molecule, first isolating 19 nor progesterone, which had four times the hormonal activity of the natural hormone but which was still inactive by mouth. From this they produced 19-nor-17α-ethinyl testosterone, which became known by the much simpler name of norethindrone, still today one of the most widely used oral contraceptive agents. The final step in production was conducted by a young undergraduate student, Luis Miramontes, later to become a prominent steroid chemist in his own right. A large man, later photographs show him towering over the relatively diminutive George Rosenkranz. Miramontes' carefully written and annotated description of the process has been recorded on slides and has become a fascinating item of display at chemistry lectures. Paradoxically, it must not be thought that the workers at Syntex had any idea of the contraceptive potential of norethindrone. This eureka-like revelation had to wait eight more years or so. What they did have was a steroid with potent progestational activity that was active when taken by mouth. Using this much more rapid Mexican extraction process, Rosenkranz, Djerassi and Miramontes applied for a patent of their discovery on 22nd November, 1951, a mere five weeks after its isolation following confirmation of its biological activity by workers at the Endocrine Laboratories of Wisconsin. The date is important, for as we shall see, it took second place to a rival product prepared at a slightly later date.

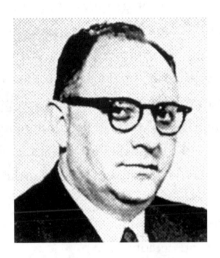

Frank Colton

One can sympathize with the undercurrent of Djerassi's barely concealed irritation in his autobiography at the later production of a nearly identical steroid by Frank Colton, concerned as he was, like most scientists, with the glory and exaltation of being first, a foible that he freely admits. He was further irritated by the subsequent knowledge that the steroid manufactured by Colton, called norethynodrel, was metabolized in the gut to form his norethindrone. Colton however, was no fly-by-night chemist. At the Mayo Foundation, during his employment there from 1949 to 1951, he had worked with Edward Kendall, who had shared the Nobel Prize for his work on the isolation of cortisone. In 1951, in a crucial switch of employment, Colton went to work as a senior research chemist for the pharmaceutical company Searle, where he synthesized nor-ethynodrel. This, too, was patented in the U.S., but not until 31st August, 1953, well more than a year after Djerassi's discovery. There were, too, financial considerations, for it was seen that each of these artificial progesterones, or progestins, as they later became known, had a high potential for marketability as treatment for gynecological disorders. It was Djerassi's further misfortune to work for Syntex, which although capable of production of enormous amounts of progesterone, had no retail organization for sale of this product or any other, including the holy grail of norethindrone. This left Syntex virtually helpless in the competition with Searle, a pharmaceutical company with a formal retail sales structure. Further, to add to Djer-assi's frustration, Gregory Pincus was now a consultant for Searle and selected norethynodrel for his animal experiments in assessing the efficacy of these new progestins.

It should be made clear, however, that neither Djerassi nor Colton had any idea that their interesting progesterone-like steroid had any value as a contraceptive.

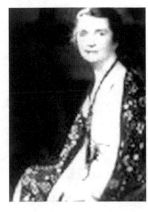

CHAPTER SIX

The Financier
Katharine Dexter McCormick

Those who think that money and fortune bring happiness will soon be disabused of the concept upon reading the biography of Katharine McCormick. She was born in 1876 into a wealthy and respected Michigan family. Indeed the Dexters could trace their ancestry all the way back to the 13th Century, to Richard De Excester appointed Lord Justice of Ireland by the then King of England. Her great-grandfather, U.S. Sen. Samuel Dexter III, was secretary of war under President John Adams. Shortly thereafter, he served as his secretary of the treasury. His son, Katharine's grandfather, Samuel William Dexter, was an honors graduate in law from Harvard University. As a cofounder of the University of Michigan in Ann Arbor, he served briefly as one of its regents from 1840-41. A gifted lawyer and entrepreneur, he established the town of Dexter, located some 15 miles from Ann Arbor, naming the town after his father. It is a reflection of the times and the high mortality from disease and childbearing that of his first two marriages neither spouse nor child survived. In his mid-30s, he was married for the third time, to 16-year-old Millicent Bond. Together they had eight children, of whom only one was a male, Wirt Dexter, later to become Katharine's father.

Wirt was born on the 25th October, 1832, at Gordon Hall in Dexter, the elegant 24-room mansion that his father had built, a structure that still stands today and used as a residence for the faculty members of the University of Michigan. As a young man, Wirt attended the University of Michigan, later transferring to Cazenovia Seminary, N.Y. from which he graduated in 1851 with a law degree. He was admitted to the Illinois bar in 1858 and married Kate Dusenberry, a childhood friend from Dexter. Sadly, Kate died in 1864 shortly after childbirth, as did her infant son. Two years later, after prolonged mourning, now in his 36th year and working for a prominent Chicago law firm, Wirt met and soon married 18-year-old Josephine Moore, a young woman of independent outlook, who was a daughter of a well-to-do farming family from Springfield, Mass. Josephine was then living in Chicago with her cousins, the Kings, while she studied for a degree in teaching. Wirt was by this time a highly successful lawyer. His reputation was further enhanced by his organizational skills in the work of rebuilding Chicago after the great fire of 1871, wherein he earned the respect and appreciation of many of the local wealthy industrialists, who in turn became his clients. In 1874, Josephine and Wirt, already with one child, the 7-year-old Samuel, chose to have a second. Two months before term, Josephine traveled to Michigan, where she took up residence at Gordon Hall under the care of Millicent, her mother-in-law, to await her confinement. Wirt and Samuel remained in Chicago during Josephine's absence.

Katharine Dexter was born on 27th August, 1875. Her birth was followed by weeklong celebrations in Chicago by her father and his friends. Later, as the child of a socially prominent and wealthy family residing in an affluent Chicago neighborhood, she grew up surrounded by servants and the trappings of social success. Josephine, an attentive but emotionally remote mother, imbued her with the importance of the Dexter heritage. She sent Katharine to a local school for girls at age 6 where Katharine excelled although remaining aloof from her fellow students. Physically attractive not only as a child but as a maturing woman, she preferred the company of her father and of her older brother, the latter her close friend and protector, to that of her peers, whom she regarded as foolish and superficial. However her circumstances changed dramatically when Wirt died suddenly of a heart attack at 58 years of age. Left as a wealthy widow and faced with the loss of social status upon her bereavement, Josephine decided to return to Massachusetts with 14-year-old Katharine in tow. There they settled in Boston on Beacon Street. Katharine, quite at loggerheads with her mother's vision of her future as an aspiring debutante, insisted on a career in science. As a compromise, Josephine registered her with a local finishing school for girls, noted for its academic excellence. There, Katharine proved an excellent student. Meantime, her adored brother, Sam, had embarked upon a legal career. Graduating from Harvard, he chose, against Josephine's wishes, to join the law firm of his deceased father in Chicago. Tall, athletic and outgoing, he had been elected class marshal in his senior undergraduate year. Admitted to the Chicago bar in May 1894, he returned to Boston to celebrate and meet up with his girlfriend, Elsie Clews, a bright sophomore at Barnard. He contracted meningitis, and with the swiftness peculiar to the disease, was dead within a few days.

The reader can well imagine the devastating effect of these losses, husband and son, father and brother, on these two women. Katharine's grief was further compounded by a loss of faith in any deity permissive of such deprivation. Her resolve to pursue an academic career was strengthened. Drawn to the scientific education at MIT, then known as Boston Tech, it took her three years to prepare for the entrance examination for, although well-educated by contemporary female standards of her time, her strengths in languages and music ill prepared her for MIT. At MIT, all the while dealing with a male-dominated culture contemptuous of female aspirations in science, and her mother's goal of having her married off to a leader of industry or law, Katharine passed the entrance examinations in September of 1899 at the age of 24. At MIT she became an all-A student, but her frequent written comments of disdain for both faculty and fellow male students did little to endear her to the MIT hierarchy.

In one of life's coincidental but epochal events, during the summer recess before entering her final year at MIT and while sojourning with her mother at an exclusive resort, she met Stanley McCormick over dinner at the resort's elegant restaurant. It was not their first meeting, for Stan had attended dance classes in Chicago where, 16 years ago, he had met, and been attracted to, Katharine, but Nettie McCormick, his domineering mother, had forbidden any pursuit of the relationship. Contemporary photographs bear witness to descriptions of him as being tall and physically attractive. In addition to being athletic, he had graduated cum laude from Princeton (1894). Further, he was a scion of the McCormick family, whose pater familias was the highly successful millionaire, Cyrus McCormick, the founder of International Harvester. Here, in the eyes of Josephine, was the ideal suitor for her daughter. But Stanley was mentally unstable. During his subsequent courtship of

Katharine, she, disturbed by some of his aberrations, broke off the relationship on at least three occasions before she finally consented to marriage. The wedding was a lavish affair that took place at the Chateau Prangins near Geneva, Switzerland, in September of 1904. The chateau was a mansion formerly owned by Joseph Napoleon and had been used by him as a summer residence. Josephine had acquired this fief during a visit to Europe with Katharine following the death of Samuel. A widely known wedding photograph of the couple shows Katharine tall, slim and lovely in her white bridal gown holding Stanley's arm, the latter handsome in his formal attire and almost a head taller than Katharine, the couple the epitome of youth and social status.

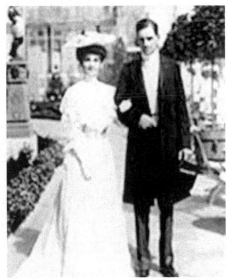

The marriage did little to stabilize Stanley's erratic behavior, exacerbated as it was by his mother's ill-concealed dissatisfaction with the match. Indeed, it is fair to speculate whether the marriage was ever consummated. Two years later, Stanley was diagnosed as schizophrenic. He spent the rest of his life as a virtual prisoner in Riven Rock, an estate owned by the McCormick family located near Santa Barbara, Calif. The saga of the McCormick family, and of Stanley in particular, is in itself a study of mental instability that we will not dwell upon. Suffice to say that the family was dominated by a tyrannical father, Cyrus, and an equally domineering, manipulative and unaffectionate mother, Nettie. We can note that, despite the intrusions and roadblocks put in her way by Nettie and her remaining children, Katharine remained loyal to the end, to her geographically isolated husband, providing, so far as the family, time and distance permitted, emotional and financial support of Stanley and his caregivers, both medical and domestic. Obstructed by distance and the machinations of the McCormick family, only rarely was she able to visit him in person. Deep divisions occurred between her and the McCormick family over the selection of his doctors and ancillary caregivers.

In her undergraduate years at MIT, Katharine McCormick had been drawn to the women's suffrage movement. At the instigation of noted suffragist Maud Wood Park, a group had been formed called the College Equal Suffrage League. Katharine had been among the first to join as the representative of women at MIT. When authorities at MIT refused permission for the group's meetings to be held on campus, the league met in Katharine's home at 393 Commonwealth. Thus began her long association with Maud Wood Park and the formation of the National American Women's Suffrage Association (NAWSA), which concluded with the passage of the 19th Amendment in August of 1920 granting women the right to vote. At one point, early in the history of the league, she was asked to be the auditor for the organization. In an intimation of things to come, Katharine personally and anonymously contributed $6,000 to sustain The Woman's Journal, the promotional magazine of the league. Among the leaders of the women's movement were Rev. Anna Howard Shaw, the president of NAWSA; Mary Ware Dennett; the fiery Emma Goldman; and of course, Margaret Sanger. However, with the passage of the constitutional amendment, NAWSA, its goal achieved, was essentially disbanded, although some of its members continued to work for women's causes by forming the League of

Women Voters. Now relieved of the demands of the organization, Katharine McCormick was free to turn her talents and abilities to a closely allied issue, the movement for liberalization of birth control.

It is recorded that Katharine's first encounter with Margaret Sanger took place in 1917, when she attended the Boston trial of a young man accused of distributing pamphlets on contraception that had been printed by Sanger. Although she and Sanger did not meet formally until some years later, Katharine had been impressed with the vigor and strength of the counter arguments presented by Margaret. In 1921, Sanger, in publicizing her upcoming American Birth Control Conference to be held at the Plaza Hotel and the Town Hall in New York, caused multiple flyers to be mailed to more than 30,000 people, among whom was Katharine McCormick. They met and almost immediately appreciated the potential synergism of the talents and abilities that each brought to the movement. More important to Sanger was Katharine's enormous wealth, for Margaret had a constant need of money to finance her political aspirations and social policies. Sanger was aggressive, a sexual libertine, mutinous, burning with devotion to her cause, whereas Katharine was educated, able but reserved, thoughtful, sexually repressed, but a proven capable administrator as evidenced by her work at NAWSA. With the coming internationalization of the birth control movement, it helped that she was fluent in both French and German. Moreover, from Sanger's point of view, Katharine McCormick not only had money, but also had a coterie of equally wealthy, similarly motivated friends.

As we have noted, the American Birth Control Conference was disrupted by the intrusion of the New York police who, at the direction of the archbishop of New York and his surrogate, Monsignor Joseph Dineen, ordered a Catholic police captain to arrest the lead speaker from the podium. With the help of Katharine, the conference was a spectacular success, not least from the wide publicity engendered by the interference of the constabulary.

In 1922, Sanger incorporated the American Birth Control League as a nonprofit organization. As anticipated, Katharine, now one of its directors, used her influence to enlist in its membership many of her wealthy associates from the now defunct NAWSA. She donated the seed money for the publication of the Birth Control Review, the propaganda organ of the League.

Katharine was scheduled as a speaker at the Annual International Birth Control Conference to be held in London on 10th July, 1922. In addition, she planned to attend the League of Nations meeting in September in Geneva as a representative of the International Women's Suffrage Association (IWSA). By dint of her fluency in French and German and her status as a scientist, she was able during her European sojourn to meet with several manufacturers of contraceptive diaphragms, ordering large numbers to be sent to Chateau Prangins, her Geneva home and the locus of her marriage to Stanley. Diaphragms, by virtue of the Comstock laws, were illegal in the United States, and in short supply. Katharine proposed to smuggle them into the States. She had the devices sewn into multiple dresses that she packed into her many traveling trunks. American customs agents, accustomed to her frequent and hitherto benign travels, were loath to question this imperious socialite, only marveling at the aura of wealth projected by the unusually excessive number of trunks in her equipage. Altogether she was able to supply 1,000 diaphragms, sufficient to meet one year's need at Sanger's new Birth Control Clinical Research office, an appellation used as a thin disguise to overcome the legal prohibitions against a birth control clinic and which was opened in 1923 staffed by Dr. Dorothy Bocker.

In anticipation of a meeting in 1927 in Geneva of the League of Nations, Margaret Sanger organized a synchronous Conference on World Population, prompted by the widespread knowledge that world population had doubled between 1800 and 1900.[10] Although Katharine provided financial help and the offer of Chateau Prangins, she had become increasingly involved in dissension with the McCormick family, principally involving the abilities and selection of Stanley's psychiatrists. The arguments became intensified when Katharine sued the McCormick family over Stanley's custody. Things came to a climax in 1929, in McCormick v. McCormick, an open trial held in Santa Barbara described by the Chicago Tribune as the trial of the decade. Each side spent enormous sums of money on lawyers, expert witnesses and court costs. Legal fees alone were estimated by the press to amount to $350,000, with an equal amount for testimony of expert witnesses. It was concluded that altogether the trial costs exceeded $1 million. Katharine failed to achieve her goal of sole custody of her husband, the judgment ending in a compromise. Emotionally drained from the trial itself, her distress was compounded by the realization that after 23 years of treatment leavened by guarded optimism on her part, she had to acknowledge that her husband's insanity was beyond effective medical care. Given descriptions of her post-trial deportment, it seems clear that Katharine went through a stage of depression.

In early 1937, the situation at Riven Rock having reached a stage of stability, Katharine renewed her acquaintance with Margaret Sanger. However, her attention was distracted by her mother's

---

10   From one billion to two billion. Currently world population exceeds 7 billion.

sudden illness. Following six months of progressive disability, on 16th November, 1937, Josephine Dexter, Katharine's mother, died at 91. Katharine had stayed in Boston with her mother during the duration of her illness. Although already wealthy on a personal level, she now became the sole inheritor of the Dexter estate, computed at $10 million, the result of her father's astute investments in Chicago real estate and, of course, the Chateau Prangins in Switzerland.

After her mother's death, Katharine joined the nascent Citizen's Committee for Planned Parenthood formed by Sanger. She had continued to contribute modest amounts of money to Sanger's American Birth Control League, but when asked for larger sums she demurred, preferring to underwrite research into more effective methods of birth control. Shortly, in 1939, she took up residence in Santa Barbara to be near Stanley, whom she visited as often as permitted by his caretakers. Thus her activities in the field of birth control consisted largely of financial support rather than direct personal involvement.

Sanger, meantime, in 1939 reunited her Clinic for Research with the American Birth Control League to form the Birth Control Federation of America. Each rival organization had sought funds from many of the same people and foundations. Moreover, the fiscal support of the Clinic for Research had become tenuous. Sensing that the furthering of her ideals required the co-option of political leaders who were, of course, almost exclusively men, male members were introduced into the organizing committee. Dr. Richard Pierson became president of the board and Dr. Kenneth Rose as national director, with the result that Sanger no longer held directive power. Over the strident objections of the female members of the committee, certain policies were changed and the organization's name changed to the Planned Parenthood Federation of America, the term "birth control" viewed as too controversial; indeed, given the tenor of the times, that was an accurate appraisal. For example, in Massachusetts, in 1942, Sanger's group, the Birth Control Federation, had written and promoted a referendum aimed at overturning Massachusetts' legal restrictions on contraception. Katharine, familiar with the political and religious environment, warned Margaret of the potential difficulties of such an initiative. The referendum, although popular with many of the electorate, was vigorously opposed by the Catholic Church, and was defeated. Under Rose, the committee chose to avoid any further religious confrontations. In the belief that the federation best represented her personal goals in the field of contraceptive research, Katharine donated $5,000 while continuing to argue her precepts on research with Rose. Her contentions were so forceful that many of the board members would absent themselves upon news of her coming! Ultimately, she made further donations conditional on promotion of research into methods of contraception.

While still in residence at Santa Barbara, there followed, on 19th January, 1947, the death of her husband, Stanley, at the age of 72. The McCormick fortune, after the death of Nettie, had been divided among the five children. As each passed on, the inheritance was divided between the survivors. Thus, at the time of Stanley's death, there remained living only his sister Anita, so that Katharine inherited an immense fortune. The Santa Barbara News Press, in an obituary written personally by Katharine, reported the value of his share of the estate at $50 million and that it paid an annual interest of more than $3 million, of which about half had gone to support the home, extensive gardens and his medical care at Riven Rock. Of this estate, Katharine inherited $35 million. Despite this huge inheritance, the payment of federal and state taxes, the sale of Riven Rock, and her divestiture of stock in International Harvester, necessarily slow in order not to disrupt the company, took many months. Nevertheless, Katharine McCormick was left an extremely wealthy woman unable, it was reported, to spend even the interest on the capital.

In Santa Barbara, although remote from the activities of the Planned Parenthood Federation, she was visited from time to time by Margaret Sanger, by then in her early 60s and in a retirement mode. In February of 1952 she advised Katharine by letter of the promising research work being conducted by Pincus at the laboratory of the Worcester Foundation for Biomedical Research. Two years previously, Sanger had met with Pincus over dinner, which had provided her with some familiarity of his work on animals. It is reported that Katharine, too, was familiar with some of his work, for it seems that she read relevant scientific journals. Moreover, she was personally acquainted with Hudson Hoagland, Pincus' sponsor and partner. In what manner her association with Hoagland came about, is not recorded. But Hoagland was a well-known researcher in mental illness, including related hormonal studies, which had probably attracted her attention, for Katharine had frequently advocated endocrine treatment for Stanley, a cause of friction with the McCormick family. There was also the geographical proximity of Worcester to Boston and his association with Katharine's alma mater MIT, where he was awarded his M.S. degree in the mid-1920s.

Sanger and McCormick kept up an intermittent communication, mostly by mail, becoming increasingly friendly to the point that they addressed their letters to each other by their first names. In January 1952, Sanger, as she prepared to leave for the Far East, had stopped at Santa Barbara and visited with McCormick. At that time they had a discussion on funding of contraceptive research.

Katharine was already contributing funds to the Planned Parenthood Federation directed by Dr. William Vogt but, as noted, had become increasingly concerned that very little of this money, if any, was being spent on research. In a note sent later to Katharine in February, Sanger mentioned Pincus' work in fertility control in rabbits. Subsequently, Hudson Hoagland met with Katharine in Boston and conducted her to the Worcester Laboratory, but she was unable to meet with Pincus as she had hoped and expected. Indeed she was quite unimpressed with what seemed to her, a rather primitive facility with only basic equipment and few workers. Notwithstanding, in a contentious meeting with the Planned Parenthood Foundation she expressed her frustration that the board had not provided Pincus with a $3,600 annual stipend. In fact the board, although highly skeptical of hormone work on rats and rabbits, and unwilling to face any public controversy over their actions in promoting the still-controversial issue of contraception, had surreptitiously provided Pincus with funds. Later in that year, Chang had been able to report to the organization some success over a prolonged period in the inhibition of ovulation in rabbits using progesterone and allied steroids. His paper, published in January of 1953, acknowledged the financial support given by PPF. However, the steroids had to be administered by injection.

Still intrigued by the work of Pincus and Chang, Sanger and McCormick had a memorable meeting with Pincus usually recorded as 8th June, 1953. Pincus and Chang and the Worcester Lab were perennially short of funds in the furthering of their research. In his autobiography, Dr. Djerassi, the steroid chemist whose laboratory in Mexico concocted and patented the first effective progestin to be used in an oral contraceptive pill, airily dismisses Katharine McCormick's contribution as that of a "wealthy philanthropist." However, with her background in biology, it is likely that McCormick had a better appreciation and greater insight into the significance than might be supposed as to what Pincus could accomplish, that is to say that the hormonal suppression of ovulation, if successful in animals, could be extrapolated to humans. It is said that she asked Pincus how much money he would require. When he responded with what he thought was an outrageous request for $250,000, unperturbed, Katharine wrote a check on the spot for $40,000, promising the balance after she had a discussion with her financial advisers or, as she put it, "her money man," this being close to the end of her financial year. Altogether, she funded Pincus' research to the tune of $2 million. Further, upon her death in 1967, she left the laboratory an additional $1 million.

Not that she was the sole source of funding. Several others such as the Dickinson Memorial Fund, the Rockefeller Foundation, and, not least, the Planned Parenthood Federation, donated money, but the contributions of McCormick far exceeded those of any other donor or even the total of that supplied by others. It is significant that Pincus dedicated his book, "The Control of Fertility," to Katharine McCormick "because of her steadfast faith in scientific inquiry and her unswerving encouragement of human dignity."

The interest and financial backing of McCormick meant a major shift in the focus of the laboratory's research. Hitherto engrossed in the investigation of fertility, chiefly through Min Chueh Chang's work on the problem of capacitation of sperm in the facilitation of penetration of the ovum, the work now switched to the means of suppression of ovulation. It was well known from the work of A.W. Makepeace in 1937 and of others that progesterone inhibited ovulation. Makepeace had used rabbits that conveniently ovulate upon coition, making it relatively easy to determine the effect of progesterone. Rats, however, have an estrus cycle rather like humans' except that it is much shorter – three to four days. Nevertheless, several investigators had demonstrated this phenomenon of suppression of ovulation with progesterone not only in the rat, but also in several other mammalian species. At first, Chang was unhappy with this change in direction, for it represented a shift from what had become almost a lifelong pursuit into a field with which he had only a passing familiarity. Nevertheless, as time passed, he became increasingly interested in the project. In 1954, under his tutelage, Robert Slechta published a paper showing that, indeed, ovulation in the rat could be suppressed not only by progesterone, but also to a lesser extent by the related hormones ethinyl testerone and 17 methyl progesterone.[11]

However, each still had to be given by injection for any consistent effect. The startling significance was that progesterone was not unique in its ability to suppress ovulation. Might other similar compounds be more effective? Of critical importance, but mentioned only casually, was that when the administration failed to prevent fertilization none of the steroids had any observable effect on the development of rat fetuses thus anticipating a major concern when birth control pills were finally developed. Further work on the rats using the new oral progestins showed a similar suppressant effect. The time was ripe for consideration of the effect on the human female.

11   Effects of progesterone and related compounds on mating and pregnancy in the rat. Slechta, Chang and Pincus. Fertility and Sterility, Vol. 5 No. 3. 1954.

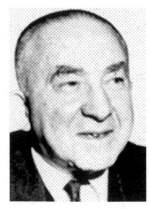

CHAPTER SEVEN

The Journalist
Dr. Earnest Gruening

Ernest Gruening is something of a peripheral figure in the advent of the Pill. Yet it was his political maneuvering in the field of Puerto Rican politics that, serendipitously, provided the environment of opportunity for the later field studies of Pincus and Rock, which we will examine in the next chapter. Born in 1877 into the family of a well-to-do and highly successful Jewish physician, he grew up speaking both English and fluent German. The latter stemmed from the birth in Prussia of his father, Emil, so that German was spoken at home as much as English and indeed was Ernest's first language. Emil Gruening, disenamored of the looming prospect of conscription service in the Prussian army and the constant, ultimately futile, military turmoil of the era, left his home country at the age of 19. Notwithstanding his opposition to military service in Prussia, upon emigration to the United States, in a seeming paradox, he shortly enlisted in the Union Army serving in the 7th New Jersey Volunteer Infantry. Ernest recalls with sentimental attachment his receipt, shortly after the death of his father, of the brass numeral 7, which his father wore on his cap for regimental identification.

With a thorough high school education in Germany, Emil had little difficulty with his medical instruction at Columbia University Medical School, underwriting its costs from fees received tutoring German, Latin, Greek and mathematics. Indeed, his earnings were sufficient to subsidize post-graduate studies in surgery of the head, eyes, ears, nose and throat in Paris, London and Berlin, where he spent time under the tutelage of several of the leading contemporary European practitioners. Returning to New York in 1870, he hung out his shingle. While the specialty of head, eyes, ears, nose and throat, or HEENT, as it became known, is no longer a single entity, having been split into ophthalmology and otorhinolaryngology, nevertheless, Emil Gruening was elected president not only of the American Otological Society, but also of the American Ophthalmological Society. In addition he became professor of ophthalmology at the New York polyclinic.

In his autobiography, Ernest Gruening recalls a blissful childhood growing up in a large home on New York's 23rd Street in the company of his four sisters, all but one older than he. Among his recollections was the highlight of his childhood, an extended family trip to Europe in June of 1894 with his mother and three of the younger sisters, where they were joined a month later by their father, Emil, and oldest sister, Rose. The family embarked upon a sightseeing tour of France until Emil and Rose returned alone to the U.S. in September.

Ernest, his mother and remaining sisters settled in Paris. The children began school in September, studying for the next year and becoming fluent in French. His father and Rose, the latter now a graduate of Vassar, returned in July of 1895. The return of Emil and Rose heralded more European traveling, specifically to Germany and Switzerland, before the family finally took a ship for home at the end of September.

Ernest's education, both formal and informal, was supervised by his father, who affected a paternal but firm interest in his pursuit of knowledge both conventional and cultural. Reading, in German and English was required, nor were he and his sisters allowed to forget their French. Emil subscribed to the illustrated weekly Mon Journal, which the children were expected to read. Ernest alone was again taken to Europe by his father in the summer of 1898. This trip included visits to museums, palaces, and whatever else was considered of educational or cultural value. To preclude any sign of favoritism, Emil returned to Europe the following year with the entire family, a vacation that Ernest describes as "rigorous" by virtue of the many side trips and multiple outdoor physical excursions. In addition, there were mandatory visits to the cultural centers of Dresden. In only one respect was Ernest unable to absorb the culture of the times, and that was in music, leading him to realize quickly that he had no aptitude for either piano or violin. However, he records that his piano teacher, after lessons were finished, would take him outdoors and point out the different constellations in the night sky, which Ernest quickly memorized.

Having completed high school education in '02 at the carefully chosen Sach's Collegiate Institute, Ernest was only 15 years old and small for his age. Thus his father deemed it too early for him to go to college and instead had him enrolled at the Hotchkiss School in Connecticut, where Ernest records his delight at the school's competitive spirit, to which he was exposed both on the sports fields and in the classroom.

Accepted into Harvard after his year at Hotchkiss, he describes, on his first days there, his feelings of exaltation. His freshman class was welcomed by a member of the senior class, a man, says Gruening, of warmth and charm, president of the Crimson, none other than Franklin Delano Roosevelt. While at Harvard, Gruening greatly enjoyed its social and cultural opportunities, particularly his proclivities for tennis, chess and bridge. It is perhaps not surprising, therefore, that he records his academic achievements as "mediocre." Nevertheless, although his father was far from insistent, it was expected that he would have a career in medicine, so Ernest entered Harvard Medical School in the fall of 1907 at the age of 20.

In his autobiography, Ernest Gruening mentions the great discoveries in medicine yet to come – sulfonamides, penicillin, the later antibiotics, insulin, but particularly those in the field of contraception. As a third-year medical student, just like Margaret Sanger, he was exposed to the dreadful overcrowding, uncontrolled fertility, malnutrition, and pervasive disease associated with the slums of South Boston. Contraception, even had there been any effective method available, he knew was strictly illegal. Moreover, any tentative initiative in that direction would have been met by the resistance of the Catholic Church and its adherents.

In an off moment of discussion with his third-year obstetrical teammate he mused on the difficulty of finding time to read. His friend, misconceiving his intent, described the means by which his uncle, a surgeon, kept up with the current medical publications by rising at 5 a.m., whereas Gruening had really wondered about the great literature of the world. Indeed, he had already begun to explore the field of journalism by publishing drama reviews in the Boston Traveler, which had been met with high praise by the newspaper's managing editor. As much as he was interested in his upcoming medical profession, Gruening wondered how he would be able to keep abreast of the national and international events that engrossed him as much as did his chosen field. Aware of a month's hiatus between the end of his third year of medical education and the start of an internship, and against the advice of his prospective employers who thought it foolish to abandon a career in medicine over the uncertainties of a newspaper career, he was accepted as a cub reporter by the Boston American. This was a Hearst publication with a reputation for "yellow" journalism, more concerned with sensationalism than the accuracy of its reports. However, Gruening mentally defended his choice by taking note of its star reporters and its unhesitating exposure of scandal, corruption and political malfeasance.

His one-month hiatus extended for more than a year, during which time he proved to be an energetic, intelligent and even wily reporter, earning rare praise from his editors. Nevertheless, he returned to medical school and completed his degree in June of 1912. But in his own words, he "had sampled the power of the press not merely to report events but to lead public opinion." This was in spite of his exposure to the sometimes-unscrupulous nature of newspapers. For example, he had noted a scurrilous and inaccurate series of articles aimed at the reputation of a respected physician who had offended a reporter and editor by blocking the reporter's access to his laboratory and shoving him out the door. There were also a number of articles lauding the leaders of outlying communities where the stories were limited to the editions published only in their area. In an "exposé," he reported on the provision of alcoholic beverages and cigarettes, solely for male guests, in an exclusive women's club, which caused a religious uproar. Of course, in the tenor of the times women were excluded from drinking alcohol or smoking in a public place.

Meantime, Ernest had met Dorothy Elizabeth Smith, whom he was to marry in 1914. Like her mother, she was a graduate of Vassar.

He took up employment with the Evening Herald, which, within three weeks was amalgamated with the Boston Traveler, a portent of the steady decline in the number of newspapers to be published over the next hundred years. In that year, 1912, he had a number of interesting assignments, including the first published interview of Helen Keller, whom had had met, courtesy of his father, at the International Congress of Otologists held at Harvard Medical School. He recorded her ability to converse with him by holding her fingers to his lips and accurately translating and replying, even when he briefly tested her by switching to German. He reported on the fatal crash of the aviatrix Harriet Quimby at the air show of that year in nearby Squantum Field. At the Democratic Convention, held in the same year in Baltimore, he had the privilege of covering Teddy Roosevelt, who had come to deliver a speech in Boston, and later, those of Howard Taft and Woodrow Wilson.

Perhaps the most significant event of the year for Gruening and for our history was the industrial strike in the Lawrence mills. The reader will recall the involvement in this affair of Margaret Sanger, who was charged with the care of the children of the strikers and of conducting them to New York, thus eliminating the responsibility of the strikers for their children, for them a major problem. Ironically, in a compassionate attempt to relieve the workers of their work burden, the legislature had passed a law reducing the workweek from 58 to not more than 54 hours. The employers responded by peremptorily reducing the wages of women and workers under the age of 16 by 30 cents per day and, in addition, refused to arbitrate. Violence ensued and in the turmoil, a female striker was shot dead. The perpetrator was unknown. However unlikely, the responsibility was ascribed to the strikers. The police arrested three of the leaders, Joseph Ettor, Arturo Giovanitti and Joseph Caruso and charged them with murder. All were Italian and therefore, as foreigners, subject to the suspicions of an unsympathetic public.

Gruening describes his sympathy for the strikers and his observations of the "crowded, foul, mill-owned tenements" and of the mills themselves. This was his introduction to what he called the realities of the industry-labor struggle. Part of the immediate problem was the public bias against the accused Italian foreign-born "anarchistic" leaders, which led to condemnatory attitudes by the press. But Gruening was also witness to the liberal clubbing of the strikers by the police, including the destruction of a reporter's camera by a well-aimed kick from a policeman, an incident alleviating somewhat the antipathetic attitude of newspaper reporters! He recorded the actions of Elizabeth Gurley "Girlie" Flynn, a woman of imposing oratorical skill, who addressed a huge worker's rally of some 15,000 on the Boston Common, adjuring them not to return to work but also to abstain from violence. A dramatic incident occurred when business executives of the American Woolen company were indicted for a conspiracy to set off explosives among the buildings of the City of Lawrence, hoping thus to incriminate the strikers. All but William Wood, bank director, multimillionaire, and leader of the group were found guilty and sentenced. Ultimately, the workers' wages were restored and the leaders exonerated.

Gruening's sisters Martha, a Smith College graduate, and Clara were active suffragists. While at Smith, Martha had been secretary

THE PEOPLE WHO MADE THE PILL

of the National College Equal Suffrage league. A meeting in support of the suffragists and their cause was held at the Straitsmouth Inn in Rockport, where the family had a vacation home, with Martha presiding and Clara as one of the two featured speakers. Ernest was happy to publish a report of the meeting, both out of filial loyalty but also because of his support for the cause of women's suffrage. This was another example of Gruening's enlightened ideas. He continued to work at the Herald, began to write some editorials, and was promoted to assistant editor.

Shortly, in 1914, his well-loved father died. Significantly, he records that Emil "left his children a priceless legacy of integrity and love for the values he embodied and cherished."

With the outbreak of World War I in August of '14, Gruening, long opposed to German militarism, assumed a strong pro-ally stance, appalled as he was by the German invasion of Belgium in violation of treaty agreements and of the brutal treatment of the Belgian populace by the German military. In October, he became managing editor of the Traveler, the Herald's subsidiary afternoon paper. His continuing compassion for the downtrodden was exemplified by his plea, denied by his seniors, for a pension for an elderly female employee of some 40 years' service. As an early member of the NAACP, he directed his editorial staff to omit ethnic descriptions of minorities involved in the news. He insisted on honest reviews of theatrical productions despite the dependence of the newspaper on their lucrative advertising revenues, which were likely to be withdrawn if the review were unfavorable. His integrity was further evidenced by his published defense of a young Jewish boy, Leo Frank, accused and condemned in Georgia in an atmosphere of virulent anti-Semitism of the rape and murder of a 14-year-old female employee of the factory where Frank was the manager. Public hysteria had been stirred by the demagogic editorial rantings of former congressman Thomas E. Watson that were published in a widely read weekly newspaper. A populist, Watson was noted for his fulminant anti-Semitism. However, it was widely thought among the more perceptive legal minds that in Frank's case there had been a grave miscarriage of justice. Gruening's journalistic defense led to the commutation of Frank's death sentence to life imprisonment. Sadly, shortly thereafter, Frank was seized from prison by a lynch mob and hanged. Watson, however, went on to become a U.S. senator, supported in large part by his populist stance in the Frank case.

In a portent of things to come, Gruening wrote an editorial critical of the Massachusetts law making it a criminal offense for a physician to prescribe birth control for a woman even where it was indicated to protect her life and health. His position was a reaction to the recent prosecution of an individual who had distributed birth control information. However, even as the presses rolled, his senior editor, suddenly aware of the article and, although sympathetic to Gruening's viewpoint, ordered the presses stopped before the edition, with his editorial, could be distributed.

Gruening finally resigned from his editorial position at the Herald over a matter of principle. The facts are worthy of delineation. Gruening, angered by the distribution of the movie "The Birth of a Nation" because of its promotion of the Ku Klux Klan and its denigration of black people, approached the mayor of Boston, James Michael Curley, suggesting that the movie be censored. Curley sympathized, but claimed he had no legal authority to do so. Nevertheless, Curley promoted a bill in the Massachusetts Legislature setting up a Board of Three Censors, which included himself, the chief judge of the Municipal Court, and Boston's chief of police. While Gruening later changed his views on censorship, Curley pre-empted the other two members of the board and arbitrarily censored productions according to his own prejudices. However, when an equally offensive film on abortion called "Where Are My Children?' was released, Curley made no move toward censorship. The Herald subsequently published an investigation proving that he had a financial interest in the production, and Curley publicly confessed to the truth of the matter. But behind the scenes other financial interests led to political maneuvering pressuring the Herald into publishing a retraction. This Gruening adamantly refused to accept, and on the day of publication of the retraction, he abruptly resigned in protest.

Gruening was quickly hired as city editor by the struggling Boston Journal So straitened were its circumstances compounded, as they were, by loss of personnel due to American intervention in World War I, that he also undertook to write its editorials strongly favoring conscription and United States participation in the war. Contrary to the strictures of his work on the Traveler, he was allowed to write editorials on birth control. He condemned in print, the harsh sentence pronounced on the young man found guilty of distributing literature on birth control, after a biased district attorney had specifically sought the case. Noting that Margaret Sanger had been dropped from a similar case, an appeal to a higher court was recommended. Gruening, in defiance of the restrictive laws, went on to publish an article on the birth control movement, noting its legality in other countries. Such was the public mood in opposition to the idea, that his newspaper lost several advertising accounts. This, and other financial problems, led to the sale of the Journal to Gruening's former employer, the Herald.

While exploring the possibility of enlistment, he was offered the position of managing editor of the New York Tribune, to whose policies Gruening had shown considerable opposition. However, the management felt that Gruening's philosophies would provide a balance to their philosophies. Gruening's reservations were overcome by the allure of being in charge of a major daily in the largest city of the nation. He accepted the appointment on condition that his contract be limited to one year. It should come as no surprise to anyone that, before the year was up, Gruening's independence of thought, his support of the cause of African Americans, his dispassionate view of the war, and the suspicion that, given his ancestry, he might be pro-German, soon led to his firing. Fortunately, he was able to defend his contract in court and was paid the balance of his salary.

He volunteered for military service, applying for training at the Field Artillery Officers' Training School in Louisville, Kentucky. In his autobiography, he recounts the amusing incident of his eye-testing where, having committed to memory his father's charts, he was able to call off all the letters down to the most minute, stunning the examining physician who thought he had "encountered a unique phenomenon in ocularity!" However, his training was forestalled by the declaration of the armistice of November '18.

Then came a journalistic challenge that later equipped him for his work in Puerto Rico. José Aymar Camprubí was a graduate of Hotchkiss and Harvard. As a native of Spain, he had an interest in improving the relationships between the United States and Hispanic countries. Toward that end, he had sought to acquire a Spanish-language newspaper and had set his sights on La Prensa (The Press), a weekly shoe-string operation. With the advice of Gruening, who had done due diligence on the operation, Camprubi purchased the facility and converted it to a daily. Camprubi went on to persuade Gruening to work for the paper not only as a journalist but also as business manager, which for Gruening was a wholly new concept. Forthwith, he had to address the basics of the mechanical problems of production, the logistics of distribution, and the acquisition of advertising revenue.

In case the reader is now convinced that Gruening was a bleeding-heart liberal, it is worth recounting his union experience at La Prensa. His printing staff knew no Spanish, so that translations from say, articles in the Associated Press, were distorted by major errors in language conversion. However, the enterprise was run as an open shop. Contrarily, there were certain advantages to hiring unionized compositers and linotypers, for many of them were fluent in Spanish and a few were bilingual, so that Gruening went ahead with this initiative. This done, there was an immediate improvement in the quality of Spanish.

However, the circulation of the newspaper, apart from the 5,500 copies sent to newsstands, was also dependent on an additional few hundred mailed copies that were bundled and mailed by a part-time worker who completed this work in an hour each night at 10 p.m. for a recompense of $18 for a six-day week. In the economy of the times, this was a nice return for his labors. But soon Gruening was approached by two representatives of the Mailer's Union, who indicated that the union rate was $35 per week. As if that were not enough, the union representatives pointed out that the work, which straddled the conventional evening and night hours, would require two mailers, or $70 per week. Finding this hard to swallow, Gruening was further confounded by the assertion that one of the two had to be paid as a foreman at $37.50 per week and that according to union rules, work performed between 5 p.m. and 11 p.m. had to be paid at a time-and-a-half rate! Gruening, in spite of threats, did an immediate about-face and withdrew from unionization. The effect was almost immediate. Delivery trucks were sabotaged and an attempt was made by union organizers to set up a competing Spanish-language newspaper, although this quickly languished. The experience greatly leavened Gruening's attitude to unions. While remaining sympathetic, he ascribed their activities as heavily responsible for the national downfall of newspapers, a situation he strongly deprecated, noting the function of the press in its support of more effective dissemination of information. But the overall significance of La Prensa for Gruening is that he became familiar with the Hispanic culture, its language, its ideas and concerns.

In May of 1920, Gruening was offered the position of managing editor of The Nation by Oswald Garrison Villard, owner, editor and son of its founder, Henry Villard, who was a former journalist and was presently a railroad owner. Seen as the flagship publication of American left-wing politics of that time, The Nation was relatively independent with a reputation for integrity. Oswald Villard's grandfather was the abolitionist William Lloyd Garrison and had been active in the formation of the NAACP in 1910, later serving as its treasurer. Gruening found agreement among the staff that the thrust of its articles would be dissent and the publication of material on "issues ignored by the daily press." Beginning in May of 1921 his name was denoted on the masthead as managing editor. The Nation took a stance against the marine invasions of Haiti, Dominican Republic and Nicaragua hitherto concealed from the public by Navy censorship, actions that had violated international law and existing treaties but were prompted by financial interests aimed at exploiting these Caribbean nations. In addition to the NAACP, the Nation took up the defense of other minorities such as the expropriation of properties owned by Japanese residents of California and the hitherto concealed pogroms in Poland revealed in the report of a British parliamentary commission chaired by Sir Stuart Samuel. It was also a strong supporter of the 19th Amendment ratified on 18th August, 1920, enfranchising the nation's women. Free trade was among its principles.

One revealing item of the times and of the Nation's stance was its support of the actions of the then-governor of North Carolina, Thomas Walter Bickett. A black man, accused of raping a white woman and later proved innocent, had been dragged from prison and lynched. One week later, three black men were jailed on accusations of assault. Bickett ordered out the National Guard to protect the suspects "at all costs," ordering guardsmen to fire on any mob intent on vigilantism, surely an order without precedent in the annals of the nation and certainly in those of a Southern state.

In the following year, 1921, after several other journalistic ventures in defense of the weak, the downtrodden and the financially exploited, came a significant event in the course of the birth control movement. This was Margaret Sanger's First American Birth Control Conference held in New York in November. Gruening had greatly admired Margaret Sanger, had met and corresponded with her even before his return to New York in 1918. He was greatly impressed by her dedication to her cause, her defiance of the restrictive state and federal laws against contraception, and her sedulous opposition to the Catholic Church. He was very much aware of her several incarcerations, her speeches, her pamphlets, and her publications of "The Woman Rebel" and Birth Control Review.

As we have already noted, the conference was held over a three-day period in an effort "to show that the conclusions attained by scientists and social authorities indicate that birth control is the first and fundamental step toward national and racial health, disarmament, world peace and the abolition of poverty." The first two days were held in the celebrated Plaza Hotel, devoted to discussions of health and social problems, overpopulation as a causative factor in war, and the legal obstacles to birth control in the United States. A private session, open only to physicians, was held where specific methods of birth control could be discussed, however few there were at that time. Gruening and his wife, Dorothy, had been invited and dutifully attended.

All went well until the third day, which was dedicated to a discussion of the topic "Birth Control, Is It Moral?" and scheduled as a mass meeting to be held at Town Hall. The discussants, as we have already noted, included Margaret Sanger and Harold Cox, an accomplished speaker, editor of the prestigious Edinburgh Review, and a former member of Parliament. Gruening, in order to secure a good seat, went early to Town Hall, which opened at 7 p.m., a full hour and a half before the scheduled talks. With the hall filled near to capacity, without introduction, a police sergeant stepped onto the stage and announced the cancellation of the meeting and requesting that the audience leave. Just as he did so, Margaret Sanger and Harold Cox arrived. On their way by taxi, Margaret had been gratified by the turnout, for they had trouble getting through the jam-packed street due to the traffic and crowd. She and Cox, accompanied by Margaret's longstanding friend Juliet Rublee, had to push their way through the crowd to the entrance, only to be stopped by two policemen, a pair among many others in the vicinity. On being told that the doors were locked, Margaret tried to call the police commissioner, but was told that he could not be reached and, frustrated on an attempt to call New York Mayor John Hylan, an opportunity presented itself so that she was able to duck past a policeman who had temporarily opened the door, and rush straight onto the platform. Starting to speak, she was almost immediately grasped by a policeman and threatened with arrest should she continue.

Anne Kennedy, Margaret's associate and editor of the Birth Control Review, had arrived earlier and told Margaret that a man had approached her as she sat on the platform to tell her that the meeting must be closed. Told that the reason was because the topic was indecent and immoral, she asked upon whose authority this was ordered. The man identified himself as Monsignor Dineen, secretary to Archbishop Hayes. Sensing resistance, the monsignor turned to Capt. Thomas Donohue of the New York Police who, in turn, insisted that the meeting be stopped. In response, Anne Kennedy wrote down, "I, Captain Donohue of the 26th precinct, at the order of Monsignor Joseph Dineen, Secretary to Archbishop Hayes, have ordered this meeting closed" and threatened to read it to the audience.

Margaret tried several more times to speak. Seeing the advantage of publicity for her cause, she persisted, for it was her motivation to be arrested, and she succeeded. Followed by a large crowd and walking after her refusal to be taken in the paddy wagon, she, Anne Kennedy and Juliet Rublee arrived at the West 47th Street police station. From there they were driven in the paddy wagon to the night court, released without bail, and ordered to appear in court on the following morning.

Gruening noted that while all the newspapers reported the incident, none made any editorial comment. Specifically, this was true of the New York Tribune, Gruening's former employer. This was despite the expressed public anger of one of the attendees, Mrs. Ogden Reid, whose husband was its editor. While the Tribune did publish letters of protest, Gruening felt that this missed the point by not condemning the action of the police, which had been ordered by a leading member of the Catholic hierarchy. The Nation did take up the editorial cudgels on behalf of Sanger and her principles, noting what it perceived as the paradox of Archbishop Hayes' intervention:

> "…The Archbishop has furnished the birth control movement with advertising worth thousands of dollars. He has given all anti-clericals definite and specific evidence of clerical interference in government and hostility to the fundamental American rights of free speech, which will be used in those anti-Catholic campaigns which The Nation has deplored."

In the view of Gruening, Hayes went on to compound his error by publicly and formally denouncing the birth control movement and by promoting Monsignor Dineen to Chancellor of the Archdiocese. Hayes' published defense has already been dealt with in Chapter Two on Margaret Sanger. Shortly he was to become Cardinal Hayes,

To further confront the tenets of Archbishop Hayes' philosophy, Gruening sought to engage the views of what he calls, with scarcely veiled humor, "another prominent interpreter of the divine purpose." An article was published in The Nation by Walter R. Inge, dean of St. Paul's Cathedral in London:

> "The control of parenthood is perhaps the most important movement in our time. It is not only universal in the civilized world, but the degree to which it is practiced is a very fair gauge of the position of that country in the scale of civilization."

Gruening notes that he continued to support the birth control movement over the next 30-odd years opposing the strictures of the law, of the Catholic Church, and of embedded social mores.

The Nation sent Gruening as an itinerant journalist to Mexico. He and Dorothy departed by sea for Vera Cruz in mid-December of 1921. In this venture, Gruening was encouraged by the promise of his friend and Harvard classmate, Richard John Walsh, editor of Collier's weekly, to publish his articles, because Collier's had a much wider circulation than The Nation.

For the government of Mexico, 1921 was a watershed between 10 years of violent revolution against the dictatorship of Porfirio Diaz and the nascent beginnings of constitutional government. Diaz had expropriated much of the land ownership from the citizenry largely at the behest of American interests, thus reducing the populace to veritable peonage. In addition, a scandal over oil had recently been exposed in The Nation in an article by John Kenneth Turner, showing that the United States had failed to recognize the current government under its president, Alvaro Obregon, because of the influence of American oil interests. Albert B. Fall, former senator from New Mexico and Secretary of the Interior in the Harding administration, conducted highly inflammatory and prejudicial hearings on the financial sufferings of American citizens at the hands of the new 1917 Mexican constitution, ensuring non recognition of the new government. It was subsequently shown that Fall had received a $100,000 bribe from the owner of two oil companies located in Mexico. Fall was tried, convicted and imprisoned for his actions. It is significant of the contemporary American attitudes to Mexico that Lanier Winslow, first secretary of the United States Embassy, while a fellow shipmate of the Gruenings, declaimed that Mexico might be a great country if it were dipped in the ocean for a half-hour until all its citizens had drowned!

Gruening had quickly befriended President Obregon by writing to him before he and Dorothy arrived in Mexico City. Obregon proved to be popular, democratic, amicable, and gifted with a sense of humor, noting that the loss of his right arm in the Battle of Trinidad rendered him more popular with the electorate in that he was seen as being less able to dip into the national treasury! Shortly after they met, Obregon provided Gruening with a letter of introduction, which, throughout Gruening's extensive travels in Mexico, opened wide doors of entry to the leaders of the new Mexican constitution and government. There can be little doubt of course, that Obregon, noting Gruening's reputation of being well-disposed to his regime and aware of the influence of The Nation in an otherwise antipathetic United States, had more than a casual interest in furthering Gruening's peregrinations.

Mexico, Gruening found, was everywhere in ferment, from the dazzling paintings of Diego Rivera to the school reforms that provided for the first time effective compulsory education. Malnutrition of Mexico's children was being countered by a school meal program of milk and rolls. There was a resurgence in the historical interest in Mexico's ethnic Indians, reflected in the restoration of some of the great architectural constructions of the pre-Columbian era such as the great pyramids of the Mayan civilization. However, with only a few outstanding exceptions, Gruening found that the states' governors, while courteous, were unprincipled politicos primarily interested in self-enrichment. One such exception was José Parres of Morelos state, who was actively engaged in agrarian reform, returning the lands expropriated by the conquistadores and the dictatorial regime of Porfirio Diaz to their original Indian owners. President Obregon had particularly insisted that Gruening visit Yucatan under the governorship of Felipe Carillo Puerto. By train to Vera Cruz and thence by ship to the Yucatan port of Progreso, Gruening arrived at Yucatan's capital of Mérida.

Carillo impressed Gruening with his enlightened reforms where, instead of expelling the landowners (hacendados) he had co-opted them into residential management, as opposed to their former absentee ownership. In the interim he reduced their size sufficiently to provide the workers with land so that they could grow food for their own use. Empowered by an honest election, even his opponent landowners grudgingly approved of his administration. Most significant for our story, one of Carillo's reforms was the establishment of a birth control clinic, the first to be legally opened in the Western Hemisphere. This was opened in Mérida under the advice of the above-mentioned Anne Kennedy, secretary to Margaret Sanger's American Birth Control League.

In March, the Gruenings, after many other Mexican explorations, returned to Mexico City and the warm hospitality extended to them by Obregon. At that time, the Southern Pacific Railroad had renewed its plans to construct a line down the Western coast of Mexico. Work had been suspended in 1914 due to the civil unrest of that time, but the plans for extension were a signal to the world that Mexico was now stable enough to pursue the venture. Needless to say, this was a powerful endorsement of Obregon's government, and the Gruenings were invited to join the president and his cabinet in a club car in a celebratory train ride to the Pacific coast. Over drinks in the presidential club car, Gruening reported to Obregon his impressions of the state of Mexico, but wondered at one point how he had been able to miss out on seeing all the bandits reportedly prevalent in the countryside. With great humor, a smiling Obregon stated that he had co-opted them all into his cabinet and that Gruening was now seated among them! He further amused Gruening by the apocryphal tale of San Antonio who, while bathing naked in a river, was tempted by the devil who placed two beautiful, young naked women near him in the stream. San Antonio immediately retreated covering his genitals with his sombrero. But the devil sent two wasps that stung San Antonio in each ear, whereupon San Antonio, in defense, clapped his hands to his ears. Then a miracle occurred – San Antonio's hat did not fall to the ground!

The story of Gruening's visit to Mexico is given to underline the integrity of his character, and his search for truth, but it also further opened his mind to Hispanic language and culture and the importance of a free press. Not that the latter was always used honestly. While compiling a book on his Mexican travels hoping to enlighten the American public on its neighbor to the south, Gruening was accused in the Chicago Tribune of being a member of a group of Bolshevik itinerants in Mexico whose aim was to align the country and the United States with Russian communism. Despite the powerful influence of the Chicago Tribune, Gruening mounted a libel action and in this was ultimately successful. Later, the Hearst newspapers published a completely false accusatory article alleging that Gruening had accepted money from Obregons's successor, President Plutarco Elías Calles, whose friendship with Gruening had resulted in his invitation to Calles' 1924 presidential inauguration. The money was to be used supposedly to foment insurrection among striking British coal miners. Once more, Gruening launched a successful libel suit, this time against the Hearst newspapers, arguably the most powerful of the contemporary news media.

While Gruening continued to take a deep interest in influencing Mexican affairs, it becomes less relevant to our story. It should be noted however, that his assessment of political characters was not always accurate. In spite of his favorable view of President Calles, based partly on Calles' later refusal to extend his term of office beyond its constitutional limits, his successors were largely his own political lackeys. Calles also mounted a rabid and unjustified attack on the Catholic Church, expelling its priests from his large home state of Sonora. The illegitimate son of an alcoholic father, he also attempted to turn the state into a "dry" one. An avowed atheist, his strong opposition to the church, which included the deprivation of the civil liberties of the clergy, led to the Cristero rebellion of 1924-26 characterized by brutal atrocities on each side. His strong support of unionization also led him to be labeled a Bolshevik by the American press. Despite a truce negotiated by then-American Ambassador Dwight Morrow (later to become father-in-law to famed aviator Charles Lindbergh.) Calles violated its terms, peremptorily executing some 500 of the Cristero leaders in addition to around 5,000 followers, often in front of their wives and children. For many years he became in effect a fascist dictator. His anti-Catholic policies went unchanged until the presidency in 1940 of Manuel Avila Camacho, a Catholic devotee.

Back in the U.S. working on his book on Mexico, Gruening was approached in the summer of 1927 by Philip Chapman, a prominent lawyer and banker in Portland, Maine, with the proposition of starting up an independent daily in competition with the city's other papers, which included the morning Press Herald, the Evening Express and the Sunday Telegram, all owned by Guy Gannett, who supported Samuel Insull, a Chicago utility tycoon. Maine produced sufficient electricity to supply its populace, but Insull, in control of the state electrical utility and in defiance of state law passed against exportation of power, wanted to distribute electricity to neighboring states. Insull was further suspected of political corruption. Thus, a newspaper was needed to counteract the local press monopoly. With more than a whiff of egotism, Gruening proposed that he alone, as editor, be permitted to determine editorial policies. To the amazement of Gruening, Chapman accepted with the minor proviso that he would be able to discuss these policies without ultimately altering them. By early October, a mere two months after Gruening's first interview with Chapman, the presses were rolling with the first edition of the Portland Evening News.

Under the aegis of free speech, it immediately and successfully defended the rights of an unpopular pacifist group to publicly air its arguments. This drew the friendly relations of the local clergy, but the tone of subsequent editorials in other newspapers led to the labeling of the pacifist organization as "pink." In fact the leaders of the pacifists were an elderly but reputable couple in their 70's with longstanding and respected views. To counteract their pacifist stance, the local opposition invited a certain Rev. Herbert Spencer Johnson of Boston to air a rebuttal. As part of his diatribe he announced that he was "so good a pacifist that I left my pulpit during the World War and went overseas. And I hold a commission as a major in the Reserve infantry." Two years later on Armistice Day, the same Rev. Johnson denounced President Herbert Hoover for his pacifism. Meantime, Gruening had discovered that Johnson had never gone overseas in the World War. Further, he had made his address clad in uniform, a violation of the articles of war, which led to apologies from his supporters who later eliminated him from their index of speakers.

Other editorial victories included the promotion of the concept of professional city management, at the time a novel idea, and the review of a murder case initially passed as an accident that had been ascribed to a fall by the local coroner. However, suspicious of the nature of the wounds on the deceased woman's head, Gruening enlisted the help of one of his teachers at Harvard, Dr. George Burgess McGrath, a medico-legal expert and then-medical examiner for Suffolk County, Massachusetts. The accident verdict was overturned and the woman's husband confessed to her murder, admitting that he had struck her with a rolling pin. He was sentenced to life imprisonment.

It is worth noting that Gruening had no particular antipathy to Catholicism. In the presidential election of 1928, his newspaper initially supported Herbert Hoover, but when his opponent, Alfred Smith, was subjected to unfair criticism because of his Catholic religion, Gruening withdrew support from both candidates. Nevertheless, Gruening was outraged by the political maneuverings of Bishop John Gregory Murray in the Maine senatorial election, where Chapman's law partner Owen Brewster, a former governor of Maine, was the Democratic Party candidate. Brewster had, in fact, little chance against the incumbent, Sen. Fred Hale, who was the heir, albeit an ineffective one, to a Republican dynasty. His father, Eugene, was a former United States senator who had been elected on no fewer than five consecutive occasions. In addition, Brewster, while governor, had offended the Insull organization by vetoing a bill passed by the Maine legislature permitting the sale of electricity out of state.

Now the controversy over electrical supply and rates came to a head. The legislature passed a bill once more permitting the export of power to neighboring states and this was signed into law by the new governor, William Tudor Gardner. However, because the vote was close, there was a proviso in the bill that the final decision be deferred to the electorate. Here the Portland Evening News ran into a major political problem. Rates for electricity were quite high in Maine because of layers of corporate bureaucracy. A tier of holding companies reached to the Insull organization in Chicago, with the each taking a portion of the profits, leading to inappropriate costs. The spider's web of linkages between the various corporate executives led to withdrawal of advertising income of the Portland Evening News so that the paper could not even be sold at the leading hotel in the capital of Augusta because its ownership was allied with Insull.

Only 10 days before the voting on the referendum, the Maine Grange, a longstanding nonpolitical organization of Maine farmers, invited Gruening to debate the issue in Richmond with Walter Wyman, one of the Insull executives. The Grange Hall was packed with farmers, but in the front rows sat many of the Insull employees and executives, besides legislators and magistrates. A skilled debater, Gruening was at first taken aback by the appearance of Wyman. Normally dressed in sartorially elegant fashion, he appeared in rough farmers' attire intent on being identified as one of the assembled crowd. In this, Wyman did have some legitimacy, in that he owned a large farm, but, given the multiplicity of his other interests, it would seem unlikely that he had anything approaching a hands-on activity on his property.

After introduction by the president of the Maine State Grange, Gruening was invited to speak on the question, "Shall Power be Exported from Maine?" Immediately, Gruening noted that as he was the opponent of the issue, the speaker for the affirmative should speak first, which caused some confusion in Wyman's ranks. After Wyman's presentation, Gruening wondered aloud why the cost of electricity in Maine was so high after Wyman had noted the dramatic increase in volume of business. He asked where the money came from that supported the heavy advertising campaign in favor of the issue, forcing an angry Wyman to blurt out that the money came from a business deal in Texas, an admission showing that a large sum of money was being expended in support of the referendum to sell power out of state. Furious, Wyman demanded that Gruening tell him and the audience the sources of his financial support, enabling Gruening to claim none other than his salary at the Press, and that no one was buying him, in contrast to the Insull group that had lavishly spent on advertising and political favors. The crowd roared its approval, for some of Insull's political lackeys were seated in the audience. Not much later the referendum was heavily defeated by more than 80,000 votes.

The Gannett Evening Express alleged that the community had been deceived by a "paid communist," but was careful to not identify Gruening by name so as to avoid a libel suit, but Gruening had the ultimate satisfaction of seeing the Insull empire collapse, including closure of Insull's Maine banks with heavy losses to stockholders and depositors estimated at $2.5 billion. Later the Federal Trade Commission investigated the entire power industry, exposing pervasive corruption. It reported on the Maine recipients of Insull monies, including the amounts received by specific individuals, to their public embarrassment. However, the voluminous reports of the Trade Commission were not made available to the general public, so Gruening went on to publish a book, "The Public Pays," synopsizing the report.

In late May of 1931, tragedy struck the Gruening family. The oldest of their three sons, Ernest Jr., age 12, known as Sonny, was attending a boarding school near Boston and contracted an ear infection, or otitis media. Properly treated with paracentesis and drainage of the eardrum by a reputable Boston otologist, Sonny returned home to be admitted to Maine General Hospital in Portland. Despite a mastoidectomy, sepsis developed, the offending organism the highly lethal streptococcus hemolyticus, and Sonny succumbed. Ironically, some 12 or so years later, the infection would have been quickly and effectively eliminated by treatment with penicillin.

Gruening continued his work as editor of the Portland Evening News, supporting the Maine gubernatorial candidate John Wilson, mayor of Bangor, in the primary against the incumbent, the patrician William Tudor Gardiner. Gruening had some specific enmity for Gardiner, who had been involved in the Insull scandal by signing into law the legislation that would have, but for the referendum, continued the high cost of electric power in the state. It seemed that Wilson's candidacy was going well up until the concluding event of the campaign, when the candidates were invited to make final statements over radio station WSCH, but when it came time for Wilson to speak, he was unavailable and could not be reached. Alas, Wilson had a long history of alcoholism, which had recently been controlled, but on this occasion he had fallen off the wagon. Although Gruening strongly suspected that some of the opposition had taken advantage of Wilson's weakness and subjected him to surreptitious temptation, proof was lacking.

The turmoil of political events of 1932 had resulted in the election to the presidency of Franklin Delano Roosevelt. Now, Gruening's former employer The Nation sought his talents. Oswald Villard had sold the publication to a group of its former editors who encouraged Gruening to join them. Much as he had enjoyed his relationship with the Portland Evening News and its owner, Chapman, the allure of New York and the opportunity to be able to influence major changes in governmental policy were so overwhelming that he accepted. Sadly, the Evening News reverted to a policy of avoiding offence and folded after four years, bemoaning the loss of his editorship.

Gruening, along with his editorial colleagues at The Nation, was a staunch admirer of Fiorello LaGuardia. In early 1933 they persuaded a reluctant LaGuardia to run for New York City mayor, nominally as a Republican, but with progressive ideas that did not sit well with the policies of the Republican Party. The election came down to a three-way competition between incumbent Mayor John O'Brien, LaGuardia, and the young, handsome Joseph V. McKee, the latter widely considered to be the likely winner and who also had the support of Democratic Party Chairman James Farley, an astute politician largely responsible for the election in 1932 of FDR. (Farley was also a first-generation Irish Catholic, but more of this later.) However, McKee had written what turned out to be a major indiscretion, an article titled "A Serious Problem," published in the May 1913 issue of the Catholic World that was virulently anti-Semitic. Gruening became aware of this, but search as he might, was at first unable to locate a copy. Either the entire issue had been excerpted from the retained and bound volumes of the Paulist Fathers, who published Catholic World, or the article had been excised. Even the libraries of such prestigious universities as Fordham, Columbia, Harvard, Boston College, Yale and Princeton, and the New York Public Library could not produce a copy. Ultimately, Gruening located a copy in the library of the Presbyterian Seminary in Princeton and made a photostat copy. He published it in The Nation, with devastating consequences to the candidacy of McKee, who had depended heavily on support from the Jewish segment of the New York voters. Thus, La Guardia was elected. According to Gruening's assertion, and few would dispute it, New York was for the next 10 years provided with an honest, effective, government, largely due to the energy and integrity of La Guardia. As a side issue, The Nation followed with an editorial critical of Farley for his support of McKee and for jeopardizing, for no foreseeable advantage, the prestige of the Roosevelt presidency.

In the early autumn of 1933, Gruening, based on his experiences in Mexico and Haiti, was asked by President Roosevelt to advise Foreign Secretary Cordell Hull on Latin American matters. Obtaining a letter of introduction, he quickly ingratiated himself with Hull, whom he described as "courteous and friendly." Hull, impressed with Gruening's experiences, invited him, on the recommendation of Roosevelt, to join him as an advisor at the forthcoming Montevideo Conference, which became known as the Seventh Inter-American Conference on Latin America. Having no political appointment and unencumbered by electoral problems, Gruening was able to interact freely not only with the American delegation but also with the various Latin American attendees. The resounding success of the conference was in many ways due to his casual interventions and diplomacy.

Gruening returned briefly to New York at the invitation of David Stern, owner of several newspapers including the venerable New York Evening Post, and was offered the post of managing editor. Once more, as in Maine, Gruening, attracted by the opportunity of reaching a wider audience than provided by The Nation, insisted on a free hand in writing editorials, and was accepted. Alas, he soon discovered that its owner was involved in a couple of political scandals, one concerning a corrupt Pennsylvania judge for whom Stern had intervened to prevent his impeachment and another involving deaths in tenement fires owned by a member of the Astor family, from whom Stern had sought financial support. Following his resignation, Gruening was asked to be a member of a commission studying Cuban affairs in which American governmental interference had occasioned the dethronement of two elected presidents, a policy that ultimately resulted in the dictatorship of Fulgencia Batista and, upon his overthrow, the dictatorship of Fidel Castro.

In the summer of 1934, Roosevelt, impressed with his work at the Montevideo conference, invited Gruening to join his administration as head of the newly formed Division of Territories and Island Possessions, under the aegis of the Department of the Interior, headed by Secretary Harold Ickes. The Division of Territories was a mishmash of several entities administered by the U.S., none of which had the imprimatur of statehood. Alaska and Hawaii, later to become full-fledged states, were represented in Congress by delegates who could speak to their problems but had no vote. The Philippines and Puerto Rico were represented by an appointed Resident Commissioner, while the Virgin Islands were without any representation. Puerto Rico had but recently been transferred from the War Department's Insular Bureau.

Gruening approached his appointment with some trepidation. He had never even visited the Philippines, Hawaii or the Virgin Islands and his familiarity with Puerto Rico was limited to a one-day visit. Given some reassurance by Roosevelt that the Philippines and Hawaii required little attention and that the Virgin Islands were an effective poorhouse, he was further perturbed by Roosevelt's description of Puerto Rico's situation as hopeless. He had also reservations regarding the role of the U.S. government as analogous to Britain's Colonial Office, anathema to Gruening's philosophical views on what constituted a proper democracy. Venturing an opinion to Roosevelt on this aspect of his appointment, he was left with the impression that Roosevelt would not be unhappy to see a resolution of this apparent contradiction of the American Constitution.

Almost immediately, Gruening, an admirer of Harold Ickes, whom he knew only by reputation, discovered that his idol was arrogant, opinionated and devious. His first conflict with Ickes arose over his recommendation of a well-qualified individual, Robert Herrick, for the post of secretary of the Virgin Islands. Ickes' administrative assistant, Ebert Burlew, brusquely accused Gruening of offering the post, contrary to Ickes' standing orders that only Ickes was to offer employment, although it had been merely a suggestion on the part of Gruening. Though he approached Ickes apologetically and made a plea for Herrick, his choice was peremptorily rejected without explanation. A later informal plea was cut short by Ickes in a curt manner, leaving Gruening with the impression that Ickes' decision was incontrovertible. He was astonished some two weeks later by a letter from Ickes stating that if he, Gruening insisted on Herrick's appointment, he would be hired as a lower grade civil servant. In the interval, Ickes had heard from a variety of prominent supporters of Herrick, among whom was Felix Frankfurter, and was altering the record to make it seem that Gruening had been responsible for obstructing Herrick's appointment. Ickes' offensive letter later went missing from the record and was replaced by one with a more congenial tone, leaving Gruening with a deep distrust of the secretary.

The appointment availed Gruening of the opportunity of accompanying Herrick to the Virgin Islands to take up his duties. He was charmed by the beauty of these as-yet impoverished islands long before their enrichment by the advent of the modern tourist industry. He worked with Herrick to improve the economy by resuscitating the sugar cane industry and the distillation of rum, which had fallen into desuetude as a consequence of prohibition. With Roosevelt's approval, the product was named Government House Rum. The alternative suggestion of Fine Distilled Rum was rejected with a laugh by Roosevelt. Under Herrick, the islands were administered efficiently during the four years from his appointment until his sudden death, his governance ultimately earning the praise of Ickes.

Gruening had found the islands' population wracked by high unemployment, malnutrition and endemic diseases such as tuberculosis, malaria and dysentery, with outbreaks of childhood diseases such as measles and whooping cough. He estimated that 25% of the population was dependent on the offices of the Red Cross for basic nutrition. Serious as they were, such ravages and infestations were but a mild rehearsal for his later dealings with Puerto Rico.

It became apparent to Gruening that of all the territories, Puerto Rico would demand the greater degree of his attention and indeed he was so instructed by Ickes. Essentially, the problems of Puerto Rico were economic but were compounded by endemic disease, a burgeoning population, and the devastation caused by not one but two hurricanes, the more destructive in September 1928 and the second in 1932. Each had destroyed the crops upon which the economy was most dependent. In order of importance, these were sugar cane, coffee and tobacco.

Culpability for the distress of the population could scarcely be laid at the door of the American Congress – quite the contrary. The Foraker Act of 1900 had limited corporate ownership of land to 500 acres, and in 1917 the Jones Act had conferred American citizenship on the Puerto Ricans. The latter act also provided for a bicameral legislature combined with limitations on American government appointees, but the Foraker Act, with the acquiescence of a compliant legislature, had been usurped by American corporations so that most of the land had become owned by large corporations, reducing the inhabitants to serfdom, while the sugar profits were shipped overseas. The problem had been compounded by the recently passed Jones-Costigan Act limiting the export of sugar to the U.S.

In March of 1933, while Puerto Rico was still under the administration of the War Department, Roosevelt had dispatched Rexford Guy Tugwell to form a committee of local leaders with the intention of formulating a report on the means of rehabilitating the island. Tugwell was one of Roosevelt's "Brain Trust." With a doctorate in economics, he had already served as a professor at the University of Washington, the American University in Paris, and Columbia University. Although the committee he formed, later known as the President's Policy Committee, made recommendations that the president accepted in principle, execution of its tenets by Gruening and his group were frustrated by bureaucratic resistance and the lack of financial support. However, in the following April of 1935, Congress passed the Emergency Relief Appropriation Act. At first, a board was proposed to administer the act, but because of objections by the Bureau of Budget, a single administrator was recommended. Roosevelt passed an executive order with the name of the administrator left blank until signed by the president. To his astonishment, Gruening's name was placed in the blank space, making him the chief of the Puerto Rican Reconstruction Administration, abbreviated to PRRA.

In addition to being perturbed by the responsibility to his two offices, he had to deal with the anger of his superior, Harold Ickes, who suspected that he had gone above his head, to the president, to request the post, either directly or through an intermediary. His responsibility was further compounded by a lack of funding, but this was corrected by news from the president on August 1st that he had segregated $35 million in funds with hope for an addition of $65 million, to a total of $100 million. Roosevelt urged a policy not only of relief, but a program of reconstruction to be carried out with dispatch. In September, Roosevelt further authorized Gruening to make loans to rural workers for the purchase of land, farm implements, and all necessary equipment, thus providing the opportunity to enforce the 500-acre limit provided for in the Foraker Act.

It now seemed to Gruening that the political stars were favorably aligned, but he had not taken countenance of the rocks and shoals of Puerto Rican politics. Without going into details, he had to deal with an unfavorable political majority in the Puerto Rican legislature, a diabolical union of the Republican and Socialist parties, which were dissimilar in philosophy but united in their goal of dividing up the spoils of political power. In this they were opposed by the Liberal party, led by the bright, well-educated and politically sophisticated Luis Muños Marin, the scion of an active political party led by his father, Luis Muños Rivera, the former resident commissioner for Puerto Rico. Gruening had his first baptism in the Puerto Rican political fires when, favorably disposed to Luis Muños Marin, he appointed as his assistants five members of the Liberal party, out of a total of six, immediately incurring the wrath of the Republican-

Socialist coalition. Further, Roosevelt appointed a new governor, Blanton Winship, to replace the monumentally incompetent Robert Gore, with no clear delineation of respective authorities. Gore, incidentally had been appointed by James Farley as a reward for his support in FDR's election to the presidency, but Gore's only qualification for governor was his Catholic religion. Fortunately, Winship proved to be an enlightened and congenial choice.

Gruening and his administration moved ahead with economic reforms, buying out the absentee sugar monopolies, arranging for dams to provide hydroelectricity, encouraging the growth of subsistence crops, planning school construction and a new campus for the University of Puerto Rico besides a school of Tropical Medicine and plans for a cement plant. Cement was expensive to import, but was deemed necessary for the replacement of hurricane-endangered wooden structures. Nor was Puerto Rican history neglected. Steps were taken to restore historic structures, foremost among which was the Casa Blanca, the fortified home of the family of Ponce de Leon, dating from 1521. In an amusing incident, when Harold Ickes visited in January of 1936, the fortifications of the house were part of his tour of inspection. The commanding officer, a known heavy drinker, was under the influence at the time and when the tour guide, a noted but slightly built professor of history remarked on the area where the Spanish had repelled the Dutch, he was seized by the commander and told that this was America and he did not want to hear about Spaniards. Later, at a lighthearted luncheon in the rain forest of El Yunque, the same commander, wrongly interpreting a speech as a threat to remove his base, threatened to return with machine guns, before he collapsed backward into the arms of his second in command and was abruptly removed on a stretcher strategically placed in anticipation of his drunken stupor.

THE PEOPLE WHO MADE THE PILL

Much as he admired Muños Marin, Gruening's faith was shaken when Marin refused to counteract an act of terrorism initiated by Pedro Albizu Campos. Campos was the illegitimate son of a prominent Puerto Rican businessman and his black house servant. Although of mixed ethnicity, Campos was considered Latin American. Educated at Harvard, his social position there, as well as that of other black undergraduates, was assured by the efforts of Gruening and associates, who counteracted the activities of Lewis Gannett, who sought restrictions on the admissions of blacks and Jews. Elected president of the Cosmopolitan Club, Campos had been well-accepted and in a fit of patriotic fervor early enlisted in the American Army during the First World War. Assigned to a black regiment and constrained by the restrictions to which they were subjected, he quickly became resentful of all that was American. Returning to Puerto Rico, he proposed the military expulsion of Americans, declaring himself president of the Republic of Puerto Rico. Unable to secure the support of undergraduates of the University of Puerto Rico, he engaged in a vituperative policy toward them, inciting a protest meeting to have him declared persona non grata. Hoping to prevent the meeting, he sent an armed group of his followers to the gathering, who were stopped by the police. Gunfire was exchanged and in the course of the action, a policeman, an innocent bystander, and four of the insurgents were killed. Campos named the chief of police, Francis Riggs, as a target for reprisal. A few days later, the unarmed Riggs, a kindly fellow, was shot dead as he left church. To the astonishment of Gruening, Muñoz Marin refused to denounce what Gruening conceived as a campaign of terrorism. He accused Muñoz Marin of being more interested in his political future than the fate of Puerto Rico, and Marin arrogantly replied that the two were inseparable. A little later he was unable to persuade Marin into, at the very least, releasing an expression of regret over the death of Riggs.

His relationship with Marin was further soured when a bill was introduced in Congress providing for a referendum on Puerto Rican independence. Marin, in spite of a tradition of public advocacy for independence, opposed the measure and went on to accuse Gruening publicly of being behind the bill. What really inflamed Marin was the proposal in the bill that, after independence, Puerto Rico would be cut off from American financial support. Confronted by Gruening that he seemed to want his cake (independence) and eat it (continue to have financial support), Muñoz declared that that was precisely his intention! Paradoxically, Gruening not only did not support the referendum, but he considered Puerto Rico ill-suited for self-government, noting the decline into dictatorship of other Latin American republics after independence.

Now, in addition to the enmity of the Puerto Rican politicos and its press, Gruening had to face the antipathy of the Catholic Church. Always interested in the philosophy of birth control and a personal advocate of its theories, besides having an acute awareness of the population surge in Puerto Rico then estimated at 1,750,000, or 540 per square mile, he engaged the interest of Right Rev, Edwin Byrne, bishop of San Juan. Early in his administration, Gruening had appointed Francis Shea as his general counsel. Shea was a 1928 Harvard Law School graduate who had functioned well in the Agriculture Adjustment Administration just prior to his resignation. His Catholic religion had been of considerable assistance in Gruening's overtures of friendship with the bishop, and he shared Gruening's views on contraception. Now Gruening, in conversations with the bishop, proposed the formation of maternal health clinics where contraceptive instruction would be given to women who had six, seven or more children. Byrne, orthodox Catholic that he was, ordinarily would not have agreed, but on condition that there would be no public advertising of the service, said he "would look the other way."

Immediately, Gruening notified the Puerto Rican health and welfare staffs of his intention to have a clinic in each municipio, limited initially to 14 of the 77 because of fiscal restrictions. His economic plans functioning well, Gruening returned to Washington to report to Congress, if not in triumph, at least confident that his programs were bearing fruit. Within a week he was handed a copy of the Catholic Review of Baltimore with a front-page article attacking the maternal clinics, reported by Rev. M.J. Conley at the behest of none other than Bishop Byrne. Even as Gruening contemplated this about-face, he received an angry phone message from James Farley, chairman of the Democratic Party, who wanted to know, "What in hell is going on in Puerto Rico?" Farley, besides having met with three Catholic bishops, drew his attention to other current Catholic publications critical of the clinics. To Farley, with Roosevelt's re-election campaign in full swing, it was critical not to offend the Church, although as it turned out, Roosevelt won in a landslide, losing in only two states. Once returned to Puerto Rico, Gruening immediately called on Bishop Byrne, who excused his reversal by saying that he had not realized Gruening would act on such a scale. Later he learned that Archbishop Hayes of New York, the same who had closed Sanger's New York conference in 1921, had telephoned his objections to Byrne.

As a consequence, Gruening immediately notified his clinic staff that they could no longer be paid with funds from PRRA. Nevertheless, so popular were the clinics with the staff that many – doctors, nurses and others – continued to work as volunteers. That might have been the end of the story and the culmination of nascent birth control clinics in Puerto Rico, but in January of 1937 a bill was introduced in the Puerto Rican legislature ending the legal restrictions on the dissemination of contraceptive materials. The lower house passed the bill and confirmation by the Senate seemed certain. Knowing this, Bishop Byrne angrily approached Gov. Blanton Winship demanding that he veto the bill. Winship was caught in a political dilemma. As an appointee and Protestant he was hesitant to sign such a bill in the face of Catholic opposition. To opponents, it would seem that a non-elected official of Protestant persuasion was imposing his religious affiliation on a Catholic country. Winship, much distressed by the situation, even with the knowledge that the bill had considerable public support, telephoned Gruening, who was in Washington, to seek his advice. Now we see Gruening at his most shrewd. Well aware that the Commissioner of Agriculture, Menendez Ramos, a staunch Catholic, was sympathetic to the bill, he advised Winship simply to take a short leave of Puerto Rico and appoint Ramos as deputy governor in his absence, confident that Ramos would sign the bill. Winship briefly demurred, feeling that he was perhaps running away from a political contretemps, although convinced of the bill's efficacy. Reassured by Gruening, he appointed Ramos as deputy governor, left for Washington, and Ramos promptly signed the bill into law!

One could admire this piece of political legerdemain or perhaps perceive it as a trifle Machiavellian, but the only serious opposition was the Catholic religious hierarchy, so that ultimately democracy prevailed. The decision is crucial to our story, for now, alone among the United States and its territories, Puerto Rico was the only place where birth control clinics were legal, thus setting the stage for the later studies of Pincus and Rock when they pursued their clinical trials of the birth control pill.

The rest is postscript. Gruening continued to deal with the maelstrom of Puerto Rican politics, complicated by further troubles with the militant nationalists. In Ponce, on Palm Sunday 17th March, 1937, the nationalists were given permission for a civil demonstration, but appeared in uniform. Their permission was countermanded by the police. Shots were exchanged and 19 people killed. To this day it is unclear who fired the first shots. Gruening took the position that the nationalists had been the first to fire, thus drawing the enmity of the Liberal party and of Muñoz Marin. Marin had already called for his resignation after Gruening had learned that his executives at PRRA had been forced to make illegal contributions to the Liberal party. Marin further interfered with Gruening's relationship with Ickes. Never trustworthy, Ickes tried to form a commission to investigate the problems in Puerto Rico, telling Gruening that this was necessary to forestall a congressional investigation, but Gruening, after an enquiry of congressmen, confirmed that no such investigation was contemplated.

In summation, Gruening noted that in the 18 months of his administration, the PRRA had made great strides in reconstruction. The program of land redistribution was in full progress. A new cement factory was providing cheap materials for replacement of hurricane-vulnerable wooden buildings. Electricity had been made available in many rural areas; 45 medical dispensaries, two hospitals and 19 health units had been built. In addition to eight new buildings being constructed for the university, the School of Tropical Medicine had been rebuilt. Most significantly for our story, of course, it could be added that contraception had been made legal.

Gruening now turned his attention to his other territorial responsibilities, in particular Alaska, where he was to become its first governor and, later, its first senator.

CHAPTER EIGHT

The Puerto Rican Field Studies

Background

Puerto Rico was acquired by the United States as an obscure trophy in the aftermath of the Spanish American War, which ended in the Treaty of Paris in 1898, ratified by Congress in the early months of 1899. Exactly what to do with this acquisition was never clear to the American government, and to this date it remains, if not uncertain, at least ill-defined. The conquest of the island, if it may be called such, involved an unexpected invasion on the southern coast met by 11 soldiers of the Spanish authority, who had expected the attack to take place in the northeast near the city of San Juan. The campaign lasted a mere 17 days with American casualties amounting to seven killed and 18 wounded. For the next 25 years the island was treated with a neglect that superficially could be called benign, but in fact, in the absence of any congressional policy, might be better defined as pernicious. The island was seen as of vague strategic importance for the protection of shipping, a notion that was enhanced with the opening of the Panama Canal in 1914. The original population, of mixed European, native, and Haitian ethnicity, had been augmented by a relatively small number of African slaves. Curiously, to visiting Americans accustomed to the racial barriers then enforced in the continental U.S, there was a confounding lack of overt racial discrimination. Most Americans who came in contact with the people, with few exceptions, regarded them with contempt as being dirty and lazy. Besides being uneducated and unhealthy, which they certainly were, they were seen to be lacking in any kind of initiative while literacy was limited to about 20% of the populace. In great part, these characteristics could be assigned to the high rate of endemic disease. Tuberculosis was rife, infectious and incurable. Diarrhea and enteritis were the commonest causes of death for infants, but adults were by no means immune. Hookworm, affecting as many as 90% of the citizenry, was rarely fatal but caused iron deficiency anemia, which in turn led to enervation, fatigue and lassitude. Malaria, also seldom lethal, was often chronic and debilitating. Thus it was small wonder that the people of Puerto Rico were seen as incorrigibly lazy. As if that were not sufficient, venereal diseases including syphilis, gonorrhea and chancre, for which there was limited therapy, were endemic. Indeed, after the first six months in Puerto Rico, a quarter of the American troops stationed there were incapacitated by one or other of these sexually transmitted diseases. As might be expected from the pervasiveness of disease, sanitation was virtually nonexistent and the water supply often contaminated. Infant mortality was as high as 250 per 1,000 births (currently in the U.S. the figure is around six per 1,000) and death in childbirth was common.

The island itself, roughly rectangular in shape, measuring 100 miles long from east to west and 35 miles from north to south, was and remains one of great beauty graced with multiple pristine beaches, an azure sea, a central mountain range running from east to west partly covered in rain forest, and a fertile if limited, coastal littoral. But this Eden suffered from some major inherent disadvantages. It had been denied any mineral wealth and the fertile agricul-

THE PUERTO RICAN FIELD STUDIES

tural area was, and is, too small to support its population. Yet at the turn of the 19th century, crops were the sole source of its economy. When the Spanish war concluded, coffee was by far the main agricultural product, with sugar a far second and tobacco an also-ran. However, coffee production was devastated by a hurricane in 1899 and never fully recovered. The island was dependent for survival not only on the import of manufactured goods but also flour, rice and hog products. Despite the embedded poverty, uneven distribution of wealth had led to the establishment of a small, but elite upper class of landowners.

Culturally, the Puerto Ricans lived in loose family arrangements, most often without the formality of marriage. Relationships between the sexes were casual and often rotational. Housing was primitive, consisting for the most part of shacks constructed of palm fronds. Wooden homes were unusual and buildings of masonry were rare. The island populace was uniformly Catholic in religion, a major factor in the turbulent controversy over the advent of birth control policies. Fecundity was high. The high birth rate was seen to be the great, perhaps the greatest, problem for public policy. In 1800 the population was estimated at 150,000 but by mid 19th century had increased to 500,000. By the time of the American invasion, it had risen to 900,000. Most residents lived in rural settlements clustered around the coastal areas, with some living in the foothills and mountainous areas. Roads were few and for the most part crude and basic, subjected to impassable mud in times of heavy rainfall. Only two cities existed at the turn of the century – Ponce on the southeast coast with 55,000, San Juan in the northeast with 43,000. Only three other population centers had more than 30,000 residents.

Immediately prior to the American invasion, Puerto Ricans were in the process of winning a major degree of independence from the Spanish crown as an autonomous province. It was anticipated that this would be accepted by the American government, with its own history of overthrow of a colonial power but such was not to be. Under the terms of the Foraker Act of 1900, the island was made a ward of the American presidency. All executive and judicial authority was embodied in a governor appointed by the president. The governor in turn was empowered to appoint his own officials. Administratively, the island remained under the jurisdiction of the American War Department until 1934. As a result, the indigenous leadership of the island was divided into those willing to cooperate with the new administration, those opposed and resistant, and a few with the vision of ultimately winning support for an increasing amount of self rule, a difference in political philosophy that persists to this day. However, with the passage of the Jones Act in 1917, the American government established a bicameral legislature. Of greater significance for the future was the granting of American citizenship to Puerto Ricans. But the early years of the administration were years of monumental ineptitude. Although well meaning in intent, the administration took little note of the need for disease control as a means of furthering improvement in the socio-economic condition of the populace. Gubernatorial appointments were given as rewards for political service. Appointees uniformly viewed the governorship as a comfortable sinecure complemented by residence in a lush tropical environment.

With the collapse of coffee production after the hurricane of 1899, the agricultural economy shifted to the production of sugar and to a lesser extent, tobacco. Initially quite successful, the sugar market collapsed in the mid-20s leading to widespread unemployment among the sugar cane workers. As a consequence, hunger and starvation became pervasive. These tribulations served only to reinforce American attitudes to the population "whose salient characteristics...are of ignorance, poverty and helplessness." Far from seeing the solution as one of economics, the overpopulation became a focal point for remedial action.

On to the political stage in 1922 came Luis Muñoz Marin, the 24-year-old son of political leader Luis Muñoz Rivera. Writing columns in New York for the newspaper La Democracia under the nom de plume of Jacinto Ortega, a Puerto Rican Spanish-language newspaper and the official organ of his father's Union Party, he presented a front-page article titled "Practical Malthusianism." His articles were noted for their acerbic wit and were widely read in Puerto Rico, more so when, a year later, his identity and political leanings became known. Living in New York he was exposed to the views of Margaret Sanger and the writings of his favorite authors, H.L. Mencken and Anatole France. While taking cognizance of the island's economic problems, he took the viewpoint, declared publicly in El Mundo, the leading newspaper of the island, that its prime problem was overpopulation. He advocated, as a solution, the adoption of the precepts of Margaret Sanger. He described the island in graphic terms as a raft adrift with a population of 1,300,000, each member struggling with his neighbor for the little food available. Of course, he invoked all the arguments for birth control still relative to this time. These were primarily economic in nature, but he also adduced the prospect of reduction of infant mortality. His arguments evoked the expected counter responses from politicians, physicians and the church. For example, one physician warned of the distortion of the endocrine balance from inhibition of pregnancy, forgetting that childless women survive at least as well as their maternal counterparts.

His sentimental view of childbearing ignored the economic burden of one more mouth to feed. The Church spokesman, Monsignor George Caruana, indicted birth control as "race suicide" and as an unforgivable mortal sin, thus pre-empting any ecclesiastic debate. In addition, Muñoz Marin was threatened with excommunication. However, he continued to excoriate the church with arguments in newspaper columns, noting for instance that a celibate clergy were prohibited from being fruitful and filling the earth as advocated in the book of Genesis.

One significant problem for Muñoz Marin was that his advocacy was contrary to article 268 of the Comstock laws of 1873, now part of the Puerto Rican legal code. As seen in Chapter One, this law rendered illegal the transportation, mailing or importation of all obscene, lewd and lascivious articles specifically encompassing all contraceptive devices or information thereupon to which we have already alluded. Specifically, teaching of contraception was punishable by up to five years in prison. In 1932, Sanger challenged the courts in *United States v. one Package Containing 120 more or less Rubber Pessaries to prevent Conception* using the argument that such interfered with the legitimate practice of medicine. And so the law was challenged in Puerto Rico by one, Dr. Lanauze Rolón, a general practitioner in Ponce, who began in 1925 by organizing the Birth Control League with the declared purpose of overturning article 268.

One might pause here to review the varied motivations of those in favor of birth control. Today, the principle is widely embraced as, at least, the emancipation of women from the burden of frequent or unwanted pregnancy with corollaries of controlling the rapid growth in world population and engendering a more healthy and economically sound family unit. But in the early 20th century, the philosophy was bound up in other philosophies that included Malthusianism which in part favored birth control as a means of improving the genetic pool of humanity by limiting the reproduction of the less-favored masses. (A confounding consequence of the theory was that, the higher up in the social strata one climbed, the more likely was the knowledge and use of contraception, so that if one accepted the theory that such were genetically better-endowed, then paradoxically, they passed on less of their exalted genomes). A further aspect was the politico-economic environment of the times. This was a mere 15 years or so after the Russian communist revolution of 1917. Many left-leaning intellectuals saw a downtrodden proletariat as the victims of rampant and oppressive capitalism. Sanger, for instance, saw the political and legal discouragement of contraception as a means by which the capitalist system maintained a superfluity of workers whose bargaining position for better working conditions was therefore reduced. In contrast, other Marxists saw the improvement in the condition of the laboring classes as leading to a reduction in their agitation for overturning the capitalist system.

Lanauze Rolón was able to co-opt some of the leading Puerto Rican citizens in the demand, by formal resolution, for abrogation of article 268, and this became their cause célèbre. Their resolution was quickly endorsed by the leading newspapers, El Mundo and the Times, each of which noted the detrimental aspects of the burgeoning growth of population. Lanauze himself, besides contributing to these articles and newspaper columns, co-opted Sanger to his cause. Sanger in turn, sent him advice on recruiting to his insurgency the leaders and intellectuals of Puerto Rican society, including as many physicians as might be supportive. In addition, Lanauze familiarized himself with the work and writings of the Dutch gynecologist Aletta

Jacobs, translating her articles into Spanish for publication in the newspapers.

Inevitably these rumblings provoked a response from the Catholic Church, which declaimed the use of contraception as immoral, predicting a loosening of sexual morals, and seeing it as a threat to the sanctity of marriage. There was also an attitude of anti-hedonism. Contraception would lead to excess of marital sexual activity comparable to gluttony. The role of sex in marriage was hotly debated as to whether it should be viewed exclusively as a means of procreation or whether its enjoyment cemented the marital union. The arguments devolved, as they still do, over the value of a rigid moral code as opposed to a pragmatic approach to intolerable social conditions. In the end of the day, Lanauze's vigorous attempt at seeking the support of public opinion failed and the Birth Control League became defunct in 1928. However, its ideas persisted and its members formed a nidus for later action.

Meantime, in the same year of 1928 another hurricane, San Felipe, struck the island, devastating its crop production, exacerbating the tenuous economy which, combined with the imminent world depression of the early 1930s, further ravaged an already overwhelmed populace. In a report issued in 1930 by the recently formed Brookings Institution the adversities of the island were once more attributed to an excess of humanity. By this time the population count had risen to 1,454,000, an increase of more than 50% in a period of less than 30 years. Misery was pervasive and, with few exceptions, uniform. Family income averaged $250 per year with 94% spent on food. The unemployment rate was 27%. The burden of disease had little changed and almost half of all deaths were due to infectious diseases including but not limited to tuberculosis, enteritis and malaria. Little attention was paid in the report to the monopolizing of the sugar industry by absentee landholders or of the effective disenfranchisement of the agricultural workers who owned neither their land nor the crops produced thereby. However, despite its flaws, which did not go uncriticized, the report of the Brookings Institution lent credence to a policy of population reduction by birth control despite the religious, cultural, legal and political barriers. A new governor, James Beverley, was appointed in January of 1932, who staunchly advocated a policy of population control, although privately holding the opinion that this would be counterproductive to the object of increasing the quality of the people. Once more, his enounced policy provoked virulent protest from the Catholic Church, no longer under the flexible leadership of pliant Spanish prelates but under the more conservative orthodoxy of the Irish branch of the church.

In a confrontational stance, a group of citizens established a new league with a more extended role beyond the exclusive provision of birth control advice. They promoted the establishment of Maternal Health Centers "to promote and propagate sexual education, especially among the poor people, relating to the medical, economic and sociological aspect of birth control and to assist in the financing of Maternal Health Centers where women might receive proper advice and instruction under medical supervision for the cure and prevention of disease so as to be able to develop strong and healthy future generations and thus avoid the grave social problems of venereal disease and dependency."

Almost immediately questions were raised as to the legitimacy of such an enterprise, given the proscriptions of article 286. There was some political dancing around the issue but a sympathetic attorney general opined that the organization might well advocate sexual temperance as a measure of birth control and that without specifics as to methods, or overt contravention of the law, the centers were within legal bounds. At any rate, the organization was granted a certificate of incorporation and the first clinic opened in San Juan on 21st. November, 1932, providing contraceptive services under the supervision of an attending physician and a registered nurse.

However, public support was lacking, religious opposition recalcitrant, and funds meager, so that the league was soon abandoned. But the population problem remained and the mere establishment of the league opened up the controversy to widespread public and political debate.

The year 1932 brought the election of Franklin Delano Roosevelt to the presidency of the United States and with it his power to appoint the governor of Puerto Rico. Such a man, he was advised by James Bourne, should be "of the highest type of intelligence and experience…a man who has courage, tact, knowledge of government and politics, and a sense of humor." Bourne was a resident of Puerto Rico, holding his position as a plant superintendent for a cannery. He had an intimate knowledge of the island's politics and economic problems. His wife, Dorothy, was active in social work and had organized a faculty of social work at the University of Puerto Rico. The Bournes had the ear of the president by virtue of having been at one time neighbors to the Roosevelt home in Hyde Park, where they had established a strong friendship with the president and his wife, Eleanor. But political considerations prevailed. At the suggestion of James Farley, one of Roosevelt's political supporters, the choice devolved on Robert H. Gore, whose sole qualification, aside from his generous support of the Roosevelt campaign, was his

Catholic religion. The choice was disastrous, both for Puerto Rico and for Gore, who soon became embroiled in a personally demoralizing political morass. He offended even his potential supporters, the prelates of the Catholic Church, to the point that the bishop of Ponce was reputed to have written to his superiors in the United States asking for his removal. Gore's political stances were seen as inimical to the interests of the church. Superficially, Gore did have one economic asset, the Federal Emergency Relief Administration (FERA), a program inaugurated in the first feverish hundred days of the new Democratic administration of 1932 that provided $3 for every $1 raised by any state or local government. Alas for Puerto Rico, its inability to raise the $1 matching fund was an insurmountable obstacle. The population had been further demoralized by a disastrous hurricane of the same year

Fortunately, the matching requirement was waived and the Puerto Rican Emergency Relief Fund (PRERA) was substituted for the FERA, with James Bourne appointed as its director. Taking a broad view of the island's problems, in a paper titled "A Constructive Plan for Puerto Rico" his advocacy was to aim at the underlying health problems of the populace advising sanitation, control of malaria, and of tuberculosis. Nor did he flinch from the problem of overpopulation, suggesting emigration, but buttressing this with a recommendation for a program of birth control noting in parenthesis, the opposition of the Catholic Church.

PRERA had an education division primarily aimed at supplementing public school teachers but in addition, providing day care centers, nursery schools and adult education, thus providing an opportunity for the introduction of courses on child rearing and marriage. Through its publication, La Rehabilitacion, the theme of birth control was subtly supported. Significantly, when Eleanor Roosevelt visited the island in March of 1934 she was accompanied by Assistant Secretary of Agriculture Rexford Tugwell who, on viewing the social and economic problems of the island, became a convert to the policy of birth control, supporting this concept in letters to Secretary of the Interior Harold Ickes and Secretary of Agriculture Henry Wallace. However, Tugwell held reservations about supplementing the population of the United States by the proposed emigration of "these people," whom he clearly despised. (There was at this time some dismay regarding the decline of the American birth rate, which reached a record low of 21.3 per 1,000 in 1932 and is currently 14 per 1,000). In a later memorandum to the president following his return to the U.S., Tugwell advised education on the knowledge and means of birth control. Tugwell went on to promote the establishment of a three-man informal committee headed by chancellor of the university, Dr. Carlos Chardón, to make recommendations. The only significant consequence of the committee's recommendations was a watershed change in the bureaucratic direction of the island's government. Puerto Rico was removed from the oversight of the War Department and shunted into the Division of Territories and Island Possessions. Besides Puerto Rico, these included Hawaii, Alaska and the Philippines but it was the intention of the government to give prime attention to the "hopeless" problems of Puerto Rico. To that end, Roosevelt appointed Dr. Ernest Gruening as the director of the new division.

As we have already seen, Gruening was an astonishingly intelligent and versatile character. Educated as a physician at Harvard, he entered a career in journalism becoming editor of the left leaning National Review. His medical training had exposed him to the problems of excess childbearing amid the scenes of poverty so familiar to Sanger. Indeed, he had been a member of the committee formed to promote and direct Sanger's turbulent and stormy First American Birth Control Conference, held in 1921 and closed by the New York Police on the orders of Patrick Hayes, the city's archbishop.

Meantime, PRERA was foundering under reduced financial support and the political opposition of the Puerto Rican government, which was composed of the coalition of the Republican and Socialist parties and sought popular political support by endorsing the views of the Catholic Church. The church vigorously opposed the birth control activities of PRERA. In April of 1935, a social worker who had been employed by PRERA journeyed to Washington, where she agitated against the use of government funds to promote family limitation. Her criticism drew the attention of John Bourke of the National Catholic Welfare Conference, who in turn wrote to President Roosevelt to protest the use in Puerto Rico of government funding to promote contraception in violation of the Comstock laws of the penal code. Despite these and other protestations by Catholic organizations, the Bournes forged ahead, setting into operation in July of 1935 a clinic devoted entirely to birth control. This clinic was placed under the supervision of Dr. Jose Belaval, a respected gynecologist. The recently established School of Tropical Medicine, directed by Dr. George Bachman, supplied the office facilities while PRERA provided staffing and supplies. The clinic, in terms of public interest, was an immediate success.

(It is interesting to record the advice and support the Bournes received from Gladys Gaylord, longstanding executive secretary of the Maternal Health Association of Cleveland, who visited Puerto Rico in June of 1935. The MHA had opened its first clinic in 1928. Formed by a group of female society leaders of Cleveland, many of whom had been educated at some of the leading American colleges, it was supported financially by Dorothy Brush, recently widowed wife of wealthy industrialist Howard Brush. In contrast to the confrontational policies of Margaret Sanger and her supporters, the MHA had quietly and with little opposition advanced the care of Cleveland's women by, among other things, giving contraceptive advice. Because of their social status, the founders were sheltered from criticism of their birth control advocacy. They made no attempt to publicize their efforts, even to the point of concealing the address of their first clinic from other than a few sympathetic physicians, relying instead entirely on word of mouth for solicitation of clientele. By co-opting many leading physicians from Western Reserve medical school, their later clinics established a high order of care to the point that many like-minded individuals from other states and Canada came to observe their methods and organizational structure. Essentially, and almost exclusively, they prescribed diaphragms for contraception and, like Katharine McCormick and Margaret Sanger's husband, Noah Slee, they smuggled this contraband into Ohio by railroad. Gladys Gaylord was much sought-after as an advisor and educator in the field of contraception. However, although her group was able to avoid controversy, its clientele over the years numbered in the hundreds, compared with the thousands of the American Birth Control League.)

Unabashed by the rising religious and political opposition, and adjusting to the gradual withdrawal of funds by PRERA, the Bournes, with funds provided by FERA, proceeded to establish an island-wide program. In this they were assisted by the promotional efforts of Dr. Belaval who, after persuasive argument, was endorsed by the Puerto Rican Medical Association, which approved of the teaching and demonstration of contraceptive methods and, in addition, methods for the sterilization of mental defectives. Gladys Gaylord made a second supportive visit in November of the same year. By the middle of 1936, 45 clinics had been established servicing more than 3,000 clients. The church, not without validity, argued that the island's problems were largely economic and population pressures were secondary to the widespread poverty. Its arguments became moot when FERA and PRERA funds were abruptly withdrawn on 15th June, 1936.

Funding was soon replaced by the Puerto Rican Reconstruction Administration (PRRA) under the direction of the redoubtable Dr. Gruening, but there was a hiatus, resulting in a difficult time as the PRRA reorganized its functions. However, in late July, PRRA asked Dr. Belaval to resuscitate the moribund birth control clinics, providing him with a budget of $250,000 by which he was able to work on an even larger scale. Gruening, ever the great persuader, met with Monsignor Byrne, bishop of San Juan, reaching an accord with him by which the bishop agreed to drop overt opposition. However, only a week after Gruening's return to Washington, the Catholic Review carried a front-page article sponsored by Byrne exposing the work of the clinics in the most virulent terms. Monsignor Byrne excused his turnabout on the grounds that he was quite unprepared for the burgeoning of the clinics and the attendant negative publicity, counter to the policies of his church to which he had, at least officially, deferred. One is left with the impression, not uncommon in public matters, of a man torn between instinct and principle. But in addition, as Gruening learned later, word had reached none other than Patrick Hayes, now cardinal of New York, who, had summarily closed down Sanger's convention of the First American Birth Control Conference at the New York City Town Hall in 1921. At that time, Gruening had strongly criticized Hayes' actions in a stinging editorial in The Nation when he was editor, so that there was considerable enmity between these two.

Worse was to follow. The altercation took place on the eve of the 1936 presidential elections, when Franklin Delano Roosevelt sought a second term of office for which he needed, if not the support, at least not the opposition of the Catholic Church. With the elections less than two months away, Gruening received a call from none other than James Farley, director at Democratic National Headquarters, demanding in no uncertain terms that Gruening desist in whatever initiatives he had taken that had given offense to the church whose leaders were now vociferous in their opposition. As a loyal Democrat, Gruening yielded to these demands. Once more, it seemed, birth control in Puerto Rico was doomed.

It was not to be so. Once more a support team of various physicians, social workers, nurses and interested philanthropic supporters regrouped. Quickly learning of the withdrawal of political and government financing, the director of the American Birth Control League, Dr. Eric Mastner, notified Dr. Clarence Gamble, wealthy scion of one of the founders of Procter & Gamble, the very successful producer of toiletries, cleaning products and items of personal hygiene. A graduate of Princeton in 1914 and of Harvard Medical School 1920, Dr. Gamble had a longtime interest in birth control. With access to a family fortune, he had little hesitation in offering his support, both personal and financial. He proposed continuing the clinics under private sponsorship. Moreover, Gamble was not only interested in the field, but also in compiling data on the efficacy of the various methods available. His longtime secretary, Phyllis Page, a graduate of Smith College, was quickly sent to Washington to meet with Dr. Gruening, from whom she learned of the political stances in

Puerto Rico and of the opposition of the Catholic Church. Gruening was scathing in his comments on the policies of the national government, alleging that "the government is pouring thousands of dollars into Puerto Rico and it's just as though they were pouring money into a sieve." He urged the immediate involvement of Page, asking only that his intercession be anonymous. Page left on the next boat for Puerto Rico. As early as 22nd November, utilizing the skeletal personnel remaining, the Associacón Pro Salud Maternal e Infantil de Puerto Rico (Maternal and Child Health Association) was organized. Members of the board included Gov. James Beverley and Dr. Belaval. The board immediately accepted the offer of the financial support extended by Dr. Clarence Gamble. With this support, three clinics opened early the following year. Diaphragms, now legal thanks to the 1936 decision of the Second Court of Appeals in New York, were paid for and imported at the direction of Dr. Gamble and were used with complementary contraceptive jelly. In addition, at an added clinic in Humacao, an alternative method using contraceptive foam and powder was employed. At yet another facility, in Lares, a combination jelly and syringe was prescribed by itinerant workers visiting patients in rural homes. At the three start-out clinics, where diaphragms were used to the point of exclusivity, the pregnancy rate fell from 104 per hundred-years exposure to 40. The statistics from the other clinics were comparable.

The association nudged the PRRA into support for the agency. With the elections over and FDR now safely installed once more as president of the United States, the attitude and political pressure of the Catholic Church became less germane. Nine additional dispensaries were opened, supported by some of the personnel paid out of PRRA funds. Although small in concept, serving only 2,217 patients in its first year, the association was able to show convincingly the effectiveness of birth control in reduction of the birth rate. But the Comstock laws remained.

With pressure from the association, legislation was introduced to overturn the Comstock laws. There were three proposed legal changes, but the two most important proposals were Law 133, which sought to overturn the law that rendered illegal the dissemination of information on contraception, and Law 136, which would empower the commissioner of health to provide birth control services via the island's public health centers. These laws were supported by a majority of the populace, led by a coterie of physicians, nurses, social workers, university professors and societal leaders. In a landmark decision, both houses of the Puerto Rican government approved the laws. There remained one potential impediment: the proposed legislation had to be signed into law by the governor, Blanton Winship, whose veto power was advocated by Bishop Byrne. A witches' stew of controversy resulted. Winship wavered. Although sympathetic to the cause, as a Protestant in a nearly uniform Catholic environment, he was reluctant to impose his views in face of the outcries of the opposition. As we have seen, in a marvelous political légère de main, Gruening advised him to leave the island on some pretext and to appoint the Deputy Gov. Rafael Menéndez in his place, who, as a Catholic, would sign the bill into law without religious criticism. And so, on 1st May, 1937, Menéndez signed the law.

(As a footnote, part of the legislation included Law 116, providing for the creation of a Eugenics Board to provide for the compulsory sterilization of mental defectives and the morally deficient, part of the Malthusian philosophy that drove the agenda of birth control reform. It was this section of the law that Menéndez used as the principle rationale for its passage. Ironically, this philosophy has since been discredited while birth control is almost uniformly accepted.)

The passage of these laws should have been the end of the battle, but the opposition fought a rearguard action. Their argument was that Puerto Rico was subject to the laws of the United States and that the liberalization flew in the face of the Comstock laws, which were still on the books of the United States code of laws. At first, prospects for countermanding this argument looked gloomy. The commissioner of health, Dr. Eduardo Garrido, was counseled first that a policy of contraception would have no effect on population pressures because smaller families would have children who would simply survive longer, an unsympathetic view indeed, but he also contended that the antagonism of the Catholic Church would be counterproductive to promotion of the welfare of the people. It was suggested that the association mount a test case with the arrest and indictment of some physicians involved in the association. The association was further dismayed by the decision of District Attorney Cecil Snyder who, while sympathetic to their cause, supported the federal statute as the law in Puerto Rico. However, he proposed that they submit, for adjudication, a number of desperate cases in need of birth control from the perspective of their health needs. Dr Gamble meantime secured the legal counsel of Morris Ernst, who had won for Sanger the keynote decision on the importation of contraceptives. This 1936 decision of the Second Court of Appeals in New York was used as a precedent affirming the right of a physician to prescribe contraception for health reasons. The decision was affirmed by U.S. District Judge Robert Cooper and issued on the 19th January, 1939. While superficially restrictive in that contraceptive advice was limited to those whose health was in danger of jeopardy from childbearing, the gate had been opened so that a liberal interpretation might be put upon "health reasons." Now, alone among the United States and its territories, Puerto Rico had standing clinics where contraceptive advice was available and legal. Here was the structure that made possible the field studies on the oral contraceptive pill.

The reader might wonder why there was not immediate enthusiasm for the support of birth control clinics, but financial support from the government of Puerto Rico varied with the political winds. The topic remained controversial and politicians, who, for the most part, abhor any controversy that might affect their electability, were, for the most part, reticent in their support. In particular, Munoz Marin, seeking election in 1948 as the first native governor of Puerto Rico not appointed by the United States, refused any overt support. Interest reignited as the population surged after World War II. Health care, and in particular public health measures, had lowered the death rate dramatically so that life expectancy soared as the birth rate supplied five times as many lives as succumbed to the ravages of increasing age. With the support of Clarence Gamble, a trial program was initiated in the form of a study group under the auspices of the newly formed Family Planning Association of Puerto Rico directed by Dr. Edris Rice Wray. Using a variety of barrier methods (foam, diaphragms, jellies and condoms), the birth rate of the subject material was halved. In an augur of what was to come, the perceptive Rice Wray wrote to Gamble in February 1956 noting that the Worcester Foundation had perfected an oral contraceptive tablet that was to be tested on the clinic clientele. Gamble declined to experiment, concerned that its use would confound his data on the effectiveness of the currently used methods.

The Trials

Where to find, in the words of Katharine McCormick, "a cage of ovulating females," was the crucial problem in the extrapolation of the experimental work of Pincus and Chang from animals to humans. Pincus visited Puerto Rico in February of 1954, ostensibly to address the Puerto Rican medical association and assorted medical students on "The Biological Synthesis and Metabolism of Steroid Hormones," but also to meet with the medical leaders of the island, specifically those workers involved in public health, to explore the possibility of studies on hormonal suppression of ovulation. When he returned to the United States he secured the agreement of Dr. John Rock on the prospect of using Puerto Rico for field trials. Each realized that large-scale trials in the United States would be nigh on impossible. Many of the states, if not bound by the Comstock laws, at least had a large proportion of individuals philosophically opposed to such research who would not hesitate to make their opposition public. In Puerto Rico, Pincus found a supportive professional environment of government officials, hospital administrators, and leaders of the medical school. He saw that a willing, if potentially tentative, research team could be formed from several American-trained doctors, which would have the advantage of eliminating language communication problems. In addition, these individuals were highly cognizant of Puerto Rico's population problems and saw these as the cause of the attendant wretched poverty.

It was known that progesterone would, in large doses, inhibit ovulation, so that initially the trials were conceived with the purpose of assessing its optimal dosage and evaluation of side effects. With the help of Dr. David Tyler, a close friend and head of the Department of Pharmacology at the University of Puerto Rico, a trial was started in March of 1955 using the voluntary services of female medical students at the university. For a variety of reasons, this first inchoate attempt collapsed. The students, busy with their studies and forthcoming examinations, were given the task of performing a large amount of self-testing, including daily temperature readings, collection of 24-hour urine specimens, daily collection of vaginal smears, and in addition were obliged to subject themselves to monthly endometrial biopsies. Out of 23 students recruited for the program, only 13 remained after a short three months. There was, in addition, less-than-sedulous oversight by the students of the experimental requirements. Attention turned to the nursing school at the San Juan City Hospital, where, despite administrative support, not a single student nurse volunteered. Another proposed trial, involving female prisoners at the Women's Correctional Institute, had to be discontinued when it encountered the objections of prisoners.

One can sense the frustration of both Pincus and Rock. Pincus' studies in animals and Rock's 1956 studies in a small number of women had provided them with convincing evidence of the effectiveness of the newer progestins in suppressing ovulation without, seemingly, causing side effects of any significance or post-treatment sequelae. Although Rock was still concerned regarding the moral question, he had rationalized this by the perception that, while oral contraception might fly in the face of church dogma, experimentation to investigate the clinical effects, without a specific contraceptive goal, was to his mind, acceptable.

Into the picture now came Dr. Edris Rice Wray. Born in Newark, N.J., in 1904 of peripatetic parents, she was educated at Vassar and acquired her medical degree transferring from Cornell to Northwestern in Chicago and graduating in 1931. Her first daughter was born in the spring of 1933 as planned, but motherhood prevented her from pursuing specialty training. Working as a general practitioner in the Chicago suburbs while raising her two daughters, Rice Wray became involved in a birth control clinic in the Chicago area primarily as a means of augmenting her income. Her exposure to the problems of the female clientele developed in her a deep sympathy for the problems of poor women saddled with large families. In 1949, divorced after 12 years of marriage and with an interest in Spanish studies but with no specialist qualification she was given the position of medical director of the Family Planning Association in Puerto Rico. After 18 months, the Puerto Rican government gave her a scholarship to attend the University of Michigan, where she attained her master's degree in public health. She returned to Puerto Rico to become director of the training center at the Department of Health's public health unit in Rio Piedras, a public housing project in the San Juan area.

There is little biographical information on this female physician,[12] but references outline her as hard-working and thorough. Each of her posts provided her with ready access to women amenable to advice on contraception. Curiously, by her own admission, Rice Wray had little knowledge of the political background of the planned parenthood movement. The names of Margaret Sanger and Katharine McCormick were familiar to her but she had never become actively involved in the removal of social, political, and legal barriers to reform. To her great irritation, her work was affected by the opposition of the Catholic Church, which she described as "awful." Raised

---

12   Biographical information was obtained from copies of a New York interview of 1987 by Ellen Chesler and James Reed when Rice Wray was 83. Copies presently in the archives of Smith College (Sophia Smith collection). Ms. Chesler is the author of the excellent biography of Margaret Sanger, "Woman of Valor."

in the Ba'Hai religion, Rice Wray was active in its promotion and was close to those of this religion in Puerto Rico. At one time, interested in the attitude of John Rock, she asked him how, as a devout Catholic, he could espouse birth control to which Rock replied, "You know what I think? I think it's none of the church's damn business."

She and Pincus met in 1954 when she had expressed her willingness to co-operate in furthering a trial of oral contraception. Pincus wrote to Edris Rice Wray in January of 1956, lauding the effect of the new progestins in suppressing ovulation, but neglecting to tell her just how few women had been exposed to them. Indeed, reviewing the history of Pincus and Rock, one sees Pincus as the aggressive pursuer of these field studies, probably out of deep-seated scientific conviction that the results of his animal studies could readily be duplicated in women, but with almost an untrammeled disregard for unseen consequences. Rock, by contrast, was the ever-cautious physician, reluctant to expose his patients to unforeseen therapeutic disaster, compounded by his moralist reservations based on his Catholicism. Pincus, with a Jewish upbringing, was far from sharing Rock's deep-seated religious beliefs. Rock had been able to overcome his religious misgivings only by viewing his investigations simply as an exploration of the effect of progestins on the human female, of which ovulation suppression just happened to be a part.

The year 1956 was a watershed year for the contraceptive pill. This was the year in which Pincus published his research on progesterone in rats and rabbits in Acta Endocrinologica, and the same year in which he and Chang published similar studies in the journal Science on rabbits using the progestins. The latter volume contained a similar, if quite brief, article by Rock on the anti-ovulatory effect of certain progestins on a series of 50 women, which he had already presented in great detail at the Spring Laurentian Conference in Quebec.

Of the two progestins, norethindrone and norethynodrel, that were used in the 50-women study, norethynodrel was chosen for the field studies in part because the former was thought to have some masculinizing effects, but mostly because the Searle drug company was willing to supply the medication in quantity.[13]

Dr. David Tyler had suggested to Pincus that he contact Dr. Edris Rice Wray who, as director of the training center in public health, was involved in the Rio Piedras slum clearance project in San Juan. This gave her access to a large number of female clientele for the study. The site had the advantage of proximity. Moreover, the residents could easily be located, residency was fairly stable, and, unlike some of the rural areas with their primitive muddy roads, the housing could be reached without difficulty. In February of 1956, Pincus met with Rice Wray and the structure of the study was formulated under the umbrella of the Family Planning Association. Rice Wray and a social worker, Iris Rodriguez, would perform the clinical work and report the data to Pincus and Rock, while the more sophisticated laboratory work, for which there were no facilities in Puerto Rico, would be sent to the Worcester Laboratories. Besides the medication, Searle provided financial support. Couples were selected on the basis of the following criteria: they already had one child, thus establishing fertility; were under 40 years of age; and for whom an additional pregnancy would not be problematic. Also excluded were those already pregnant or who had undergone sterilization. This surgical procedure was then a popular method of birth control on the island, but because of expense, was for many quite unaffordable.

---

13   The choice was ultimately shown to be academic, for norethynodrel, after ingestion, is converted to norethindrone.

By late March, 100 eligible women had been selected, along with the necessary 125 controls matched in age and childbearing history. The study group was given careful instructions, which essentially match those of modern times, except that the pill contained a hefty 20 milligrams of norethynodrel, or about 60 times the modern dose. The pill was to be taken daily, beginning five days after the onset of menses, and continued for 20 days. If forgotten on any one day, the dose was to be doubled on the next. The dose was also to be doubled should there be any intermenstrual bleeding. Rice Wray found little reticence among her study group. Indeed, she reported that enthusiasm ran high so that she had no difficulty with recruitment and that the number of applicants far exceeded her needs.

But there were problems. It would be scarcely surprising that such an enterprise would escape public notice. Word leaked out to the local newspapers. No later than April, questions were asked of Dr. Juan Pons, secretary of health, by a local reporter, of the propriety of using public health facilities and personnel for an experiment on birth control. Rice Wray defended the study by stating, correctly, that she was supported by private funds, that her work was separated from her governmental duties, and that clientele were neither seen nor examined in public health centers. In fact, they were seen in their homes, where they were instructed in the method of use of the oral contraceptive. A few were seen at the offices of the Family Planning Association for such items.

While satisfied with Rice Wray's defense, the attendant publicity led some women to discontinue medication. Though these were easily replaced by other willing, enthusiastic clients, disturbing side effects were seen: nausea, vomiting, breast enlargement and tenderness, dizziness and headache.[14] By June 30th, of the original 211, a hundred had dropped out; some were already pregnant[15] at the outset and some had had a sterilization procedure.

Pincus and the director of medical research at Searle were duly impressed by the available data when they visited Puerto Rico in the fall of '56, but Rock still demurred. While it was clear that the pill was an effective contraceptive, he had reservations over questions of safety and long-term side effects. These concerns have already been alluded to. Who knew what the long-term effects might be on future fertility, on promotion of cancerous growths, or on general health? Meantime, in late 1956 Rice Wray resigned, citing continuing difficulties with Dr. Pons, secretary of health, but not before compiling her data. It is worth noting these data, for they formed the basis for FDA approval in June of the following year, 1957.

Of 221 women exposed to the pill, a mere 17 had become pregnant, largely due to failure to take the medication as prescribed. In a total of 47 woman-years of consistent use, there was not a single pregnancy. (Without contraception, the pregnancy rate in fertile Puerto Rican women was 65 per 100 per year.) Half of the original 109 dropped out, many by reason of side effects, which Rice Wray concluded made the method unacceptable. Here is her analysis of withdrawn clients:

---

14   These symptoms are still recognized today, even with the greatly reduced dosage, but are much less frequent. Pincus attributed them to "contamination" of the pill by a potent estrogen soon identified as mestranol. However, removal of the mestranol led to an increase in intermenstrual bleeding, so the mestranol was replaced. Today, many oral contraceptive pills still contain a small amount of estrogen, either mestranol or ethynodiol diacetate.

15   The reader should be aware that early detection of pregnancy, now possible by a simple in-office procedure, even before the first missed period, was much less practical in the 1950s. Testing was cumbersome and expensive, relying as it did on a variety of biological tests on rabbits, frogs and toads.

Reasons	Number (109)	Percentage
Pregnancies	25 (incl. 8 pregnant before starting o/c)	22.9/ 221
Reaction (nausea etc.)	25	22.9
Sterilized	15	13.9
Moved away	12	11.0
Husband opposed	9	8.3
Separated	6	5.1
Not interested	6	5.1
Physician's advice	6	5.1
Religion	3	2.7
Bleeding	2	1.8

And her analysis of reactions:

Total no. of subjects on Enovid (original 106 plus 115 added later)	221
Total having reactions	38
Percentage having reactions	17.43

Symptoms:	No. out of 38 complaining	Percentage
Dizziness	29	76.12
Nausea	26	68.16
Headache	18	47.14
Vomiting	17	44.28
Abdominal pain	9	23.26
Weakness	7	18.16
Diarrhea	1	2.24

But these symptoms, for the most part, resolved with continued use:

Onset of reaction	Number of patients
At start	13
1st month	3
2rd month	3
4th month	5
5th month	5
6th month	3
7th month	5
8th month	1

It was also noted that in at least two patients, the symptom of dysmenorrhea was resolved and a third patient was relieved of her menorrhagia (heavy menstrual bleeding).

Rice Wray was succeeded by Dr. Manuel Paniagua, who refuted Rice Wray's conclusion of unacceptability by virtue of troublesome side effects, noting that these side effects were reduced in number and intensity the longer the medication was continued, a fact still apparent today. Additional research concluded that the side effects were due, at least in part, to the instructions given to the women of Puerto Rico which advised them of the likely symptoms whereas it was noted that the women in the United States, told of little or none of the possible side effects, had many fewer complaints. Pejorative comments on the hysterical personalities of Puerto Rican women were put to rest when they later were not advised of possible side effects, but had to recognize these spontaneously, so their complaints were on a level with their American sisters.

Pincus and Panagua devised a simple but quite unethical experiment in which one of three groups of women was given the contraceptive pill with the usual warnings of side effects, a second group was given a placebo while using alternate methods of birth control, but still with the customary warnings, and the third group was given the contraceptive pill without warnings. The two first groups given warnings had only a modest difference in complaints despite the use of placebo, while the third group, given no warnings, had a much reduced incidence of complaints. It is not recorded how many of the placebo group inadvertently became pregnant using less efficacious methods! However, the study did provide convincing evidence of the power of suggestion.

Rice Wray's data were presented at a symposium sponsored by Searle on 23rd January, 1957, on 19-nor progestational steroids and attended by Rock, Pincus and others who gave presentations on one or another aspect of the theories and results of a variety of laboratory and clinical trials. Among the presentations was one by Dr. Anna L. Southam showing a reduction in menorrhagia in a small group of women and another by Dr. C. Herman Weinberg showing a marked reduction in the symptom of dysmenorrhea among 13 pill users. These results were published by Searle in a small, obscure booklet titled "Proceedings of a Symposium on 19-nor Progestational Steroids."

In addition to the Puerto Rican field study, a contemporary study had started in Los Angeles in June of 1956 under the direction of Dr. Edward T. Tyler. Another study had begun in Haiti, promoted by Pincus. Thus, in 1957 the investigators were able to present a total of 600 cases to the FDA, which approved the use of the Enovid 10-milligram pill on 10th June, 1957 – but not for contraception! The approval was for correction of menstrual disorders such as dysmenorrhea and menorrhagia. But the contraceptive effect became widely known among women, so that by mid-1959 it was estimated that half a million women were taking the medication, far more than the estimate of the incidence of menstrual disorders. Of course, it helped that the drug advisory included a warning that women taking the medication would be unable to become pregnant. It is noted that Katharine McCormick was delighted. With commendable foresight, she saw that its use for menstrual disorders "is leading inevitably to its use against pregnancy."

Clarence Gamble, always interested in contraceptive trials, in January of 1956 explored the possibility of further studies in

Humacao, recruiting the services of Adaline Pendleton Satterthwaite. Yet another exceptional female physician, Dr. Satterthwaite had graduated magna cum laude from Pomona College then earned a medical degree from University of California. Satterthwaite lived in Puerto Rico from 1952 to 1967 after a long residence in China, where she and her husband, William Satterthwaite, had worked as medical missionaries. Like many others, she was motivated to help women who had more children than they could support. The project got under way in April of 1956. She gathered her birth control data in the rural location of Humacoa, about 15 miles from San Juan. Not only were the trials successful, but the volume of clientele exceeded that of the Rio Piedras project, limited only by Searle's supply of the progestin now marketed under the name of Enovid, thus enabling Satterthwaite to vary the dosage for tests of efficacy.

Final approval of the pill as a means of contraception had to wait three more years. Even so, despite the accumulating evidence of effectiveness and safety, Rock had difficulty with the Food and Drug Administration (FDA). This government authority, at the time of application in 1959, was essentially charged by the 1938 Food, Drug and Cosmetic Act with ensuring the safety of any proposed drug and the *prohibition of false therapeutic claims.*[16]

So far as the pill was concerned, the problem of safety was hardly an issue or, at least, should not have been. Rock and Pincus by 1959 had ample data showing freedom from serious side effects or complications from its use. They had a series of cases of 897 women exposed to the pill for a total of more than 10,000 cycles. Nevertheless, the whole idea of contraception was still embedded in the

---

16   See U.S. Food and Drug Administration – History of the FDA. This would seem to refute DeFelice's rationalization that drugs need only be safe.

social mores of the time so that it was hardly even a topic fit for discussion in polite society. Even Searle was hesitant. The allure of immense profits from a drug that had to be taken each day by a huge number of potential clientele had to be balanced against the putative negative public reaction, which, in turn, might lead to a boycott of Searle's other products despite the company's shining reputation for high ethical standards. It faced competitive pressure from the Syntex product Norlutin containing Djerassi's norethindrone, which had meantime been approved under license to Parke-Davis for the same menstrual dysfunctions as Enovid, even if Parke-Davis, located in heavily Catholic Detroit and with a devout Catholic as company president, was quite opposed to marketing its product as a contraceptive. Indeed, it is recorded that the president of Parke-Davis contacted John Searle, making his philosophy known in no uncertain terms, telling Searle that he was "crazy" to contemplate such an action. So adamant was his stance that Parke-Davis later refused to release its animal studies to Ortho, the company that later released norethindrone as the contraceptive Ortho-novum, thus delaying the marketing of its product until 1962 – two years after FDA approval of oral contraception. Further proof of the negativity of the drug companies was provided by the earlier refusal of Pfizer to Syntex's offer of providing norethindrone. Pfizer's president, likewise Catholic, wanted nothing even remotely to do with a drug that was a potential contraceptive. Even Goodyear Rubber, a principle manufacturer of condoms, had carefully distanced itself from this aspect of its business.

But at Searle, Rock and Pincus had found staunch allies in John Searle, cautious but judicious, and Irwin C. Winter ("Icy" Winter, as he was known), director of research, each solidly in support of seeking FDA approval for release as a contraceptive. John Searle, descendant of founder Gideon Searle, had long taken an interest in world population growth, contributing a great deal of financial support to the population control movement. Neither was I.C. Winter any stranger to this problem. Two of his sisters were medical missionaries in India, which had provided him with an intimate knowledge of the poverty and destitution prevalent in the Indian subcontinent attributable to unconstrained growth of population. It was in large part from his friendship with the medical director of the FDA that initial approval was obtained in 1957.

Pincus, as always restless and impatient, saw no reason for further testing simply to appease the recalcitrance of the FDA bureaucracy. He was already on the world lecture circuit, courtesy of funds from Katharine McCormick, announcing the imminence of the birth control pill.

The concerns of the management of Searle regarding public reaction to release of a contraceptive were allayed by a couple of public relations trial balloons. Two articles in the Saturday Evening Post and another in the Reader's Digest carried the news that the pill, now released for menstrual disorders, was also a promising birth control agent. It is not recorded that the management awaited the outcome with bated breath, but it must have had at least some trepidation over the public reaction. There was none!

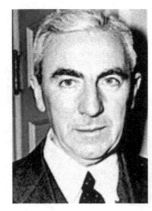

CHAPTER NINE

The Gynecologist
Dr. John Rock

Like Margaret Sanger, John Rock was born into a Catholic family. Like Sanger, he came to reject the church but, in contradistinction to Sanger's precipitate and rebellious religious apostasy, Rock's ultimate dissent was more akin to the sigh of a rejected suitor. It was a mark of his character that he was able finally and reluctantly to divorce himself from the tenets of his much-loved church in favor of cold, hard, scientific facts.

John Rock was born on 24th March, 1890, in the small town of Marlborough, Massachusetts, the fourth child of Frank and Anne Rock, who were second-generation Irish immigrants. His birth was followed almost immediately by that of his twin sister, Nell, whom he always held in much affection. His grandfather, also named John Rock, had emigrated around 1847 from County Armagh in Northern Ireland, a county of Ulster. This was the time of the terrible Irish potato famine. Frank, John's father, was married to Anne Jane Murphy. The family was, to varying degrees, devoutly Catholic, as were the majority of the inhabitants of Marlborough. However, it is to be noted that despite the prohibitions of the Catholic Church against contraception, the Rock children were evenly spaced two years apart.

With the exception of the Protestant minority, most Marlborough inhabitants were of limited means. However, as a result of Grandfather John's entrepreneurial spirit, the Rock family was relatively prosperous. Although Grandfather John had purchased a fair amount of land and other property, it was so heavily mortgaged that Frank Rock and his brother John had to leave school at an early age in order to service the mortgage debt, which they did by virtue of hard work and genial personality. In this they were moderately successful. They first established the local drugstore where, in addition to conventional pharmaceuticals, certain strong medicines of high alcoholic content could be purchased. The business acumen of the brothers led in succession to the establishment of a saloon, followed later by a theater suitable for acts by troupes of travelling companies. Subsequently this became a movie theater. They also ran a small stable of racehorses. It is said that these influences resulted in John Rock's main interests in life: medicine, the dramatic arts and liquor!

Unlike his older brothers Charles and Henry, who shared their father's love of sports, card playing and serious drinking, John was reserved almost to the point of effeminacy, acquiring the nickname of Sissy. Indeed, his brothers were appalled when, with his sister, Nell, he took sewing lessons. Although he later became a star track athlete, he eschewed the rougher team games espoused by his brothers and their robust and vigorous friends. He sought for companions the more sophisticated youths of the local Protestant families. He admired not only their manners but was attracted by their relative affluence so that one has the sense that John Rock, even as a child, was not to be satisfied with the allure of a bucolic life in Marlborough or its paucity of intellectual challenges. This became a pattern in his life, such that a caustic observer might have accused him of social climbing. Indeed, Rock and Nell learned piano and joined an exclusive group of local amateur performers where, once accepted, Rock tried to exclude additional members who, in his view, were less desirable.

His relationship with his church was strong. He was given to religious readings and compulsive daily church attendance even in his early years. He would proselytize his Protestant friends into joining him at services in the belief that he was presenting them with something good and wonderful. He tried, without success, to persuade a tolerant but skeptical father into a more sincere embrace of church conventions and religious observations.

It is a mark of John Rock's independence of mind that, after finishing his first year of high school, he sought his father's permission to attend the Boston High School of Business some 35 miles from Marlborough and which, by virtue of this distance, required residence at the school. Although John Rock had heard of the school from friends at summer camp, he could hardly have inquired thoroughly into its reputation. Indeed, while it is now a prominent Boston high school with a tradition of preparation for business careers, at the time of Rock's application, it had been established only the year before, in 1906. Further, its educational format was more in line for training in secretarial work rather than a formal business career. However, it was John Rock's aspiration to enter into the world of commerce for which, as more judicious observers knew and which for him eventually became a revelation, he was ill-suited. Nevertheless, he moved in with his father's business friends, the Flynns, whose wife he came to dislike.[17] As a result of his dislike, he exerted his independence once more, peremptorily moving to a boarding house recommended by a fellow student and going on to graduate in 1909. While at school, his athletic abilities blossomed into memberships on the track and swimming teams, resulting in his election to president of the athletic association.

Upon completion of school, and with his father financially constrained by the town of Marlborough going dry, Rock entered the business world but soon, after two or three benighted attempts at filling ill-suited posts, he was quickly disabused of any illusions he harbored regarding his supposed inherent business acumen. This would be but a footnote in Rock's career but for the fact that his first job was employment by the United Fruit Co. as timekeeper in a banana plantation in Guatemala. Here he became acquainted with the local physician, Neil McPhail, a Scottish graduate whose proclivities for the local saloons and bordellos seemed not to distract greatly from his attentions to his patients. Indeed, McPhail was later to establish a local hospital that earned, for him and itself, an international reputation for the diagnosis and treatment of tropical diseases. And so, as a relief from the miseries of an insufferably hot and humid climate, churlish overseers, and unrest among the ill-paid and ill-treated Jamaican workers, Rock sought McPhail's company. The good doctor, besides introducing Rock into the practice of medicine also facilitated his loss of virginity with one of the local prostitutes. McPhail let him assist with surgery; in the process the younger man learned a little about anesthesia and how to tie surgical knots. Thus was established a lifelong friendship, offset only somewhat later when

---

17   It is speculated that Delia Flynn became the mistress of Frank Rock. After the death of Ann, Frank's wife, he married the widow Delia, who was disliked not only by John but by all of his siblings.

it became clear to McPhail that Rock was not interested in joining him in practice. Rock, taking the side of the workers in a dispute over the arbitrary reduction in their wages, was fired after a difficult nine months in the tropics, having tolerated even this short period out of loyalty to his father, who desperately needed the cash remittances from John's well-paid job. However, his brief but intense association with McPhail determined his decision to pursue a medical career.

Credited with an extra year at business school although not officially due to graduate until 1915, to the delight of both himself and his family, he wrote and passed the Harvard College entrance exams and was accepted into Harvard Medical School in 1914 despite only average grades. His father, but mostly his brother Charlie, were happy to pay the $300 annual fees. At the college he won his letter in track each year, attended Mass frequently if sporadically, gave his energies into resuscitation of the nearly defunct Newman club, a Catholic organization whose goals were enhanced spirituality, community service and collegiality, and also participated in the Hasty Pudding presentations.[18] He befriended Sherman "Shermie" Thorndike, grandson of Gen. Tecumseh Sherman, later to become his brother-in-law when he married Shermie's sister Ann. Doubtless, it was Shermie who facilitated his membership of the Institute of 1770 club, a significant step up in the stuffy Harvard social order of the times, where there was a hierarchy of clubs, the topmost limited to all but a few of the sons of Boston's most elite. Despite the exigencies of World War I and patriotic pressure to enlist, Rock, along with most of his classmates, was persuaded by wiser heads into completing his degree, the most forceful argument being that the military had more need of qualified doctors than raw medical students. And so he

18   This was related to a journalist, probably Loretta McLaughlin, but the Harvard record does not confirm these activities.

and his class graduated in 1918. It is one of the paradoxes of Rock's subsequent luminous career that his grades at Harvard Medical School were no better than mediocre.

In July 1918 he entered a year of straight internship in surgery. In January of 1919 the family was devastated by the sudden death of their mother, Ann Rock. His father, Frank, and twin sister, Nell, the latter without any marketable skills, moved in with John. Meantime, Neil McPhail was pressuring him into joining his practice in Guatemala, where he had by then built his hospital in Quirigua and led a well-qualified staff of physicians from Edinburgh and Johns Hopkins. Tempted by the offer and the opportunity to escape family entanglements, he nevertheless decided against this course, much to McPhail's lasting irritation.

Profoundly influenced by the then-novel sexual theories of Sigmund Freud, Rock was at first attracted to a career in psychiatry, but was discouraged by the length of formal training. Instead he embarked on residency training in gynecology at the Free Hospital for Women. After a year he had a brief four months training at Massachusetts General Hospital in genitor-urinary surgery, finally going into six months residency in obstetrics and gynecology in July 1920 at Boston Lying-In Hospital. Tasked as part of his responsibilities with domiciliary obstetrics, like his contemporaries Sanger and Gruening, he was appalled by the consequences of multiple childbearing, the pervasive ignorance of sexual matters, and the horrors of preventable obstetrical disasters. Finishing residency training in January of 1921, he took a post as assistant surgeon at Massachusetts General.

Just as all seemed set for a settled family future, Frank Rock announced his intention to marry Delia Flynn, now widowed and 15 years his junior. John's dislike for Delia extended to loathing, a sentiment shared by his siblings. Older brother Charlie, to whom he was close and would become closer over the years, soon at 36 years old finally married a longstanding girlfriend. Even the unattractive and little-educated Nell married within a few months. Thus Rock became somewhat isolated from his family.

Appointed in 1922 as an assistant in obstetrics at the Harvard Medical School, in 1924 he was offered the opportunity to reactivate the infertility clinic at Massachusetts General. Thus began his lifetime interest in this field. A similar clinic at the Free Hospital for Women was established in the same year. While infertility became the topic to which he devoted most of his research, it is perhaps the great irony of the life of this great protagonist of birth control that his research was directed towards promoting fertility rather than its suppression. At this point, with a reasonably secure income, he embarked on matrimony.

Rock's proclivity for social climbing was further suggested when, with some income from his post, he chose as his bride Ann Thorndike, the daughter of a Boston Brahmin family. Ann Thorndike's maternal grandfather was Gen. Tecumseh Sherman and she was the daughter of Paul Thorndike a prominent genito-urinary surgeon. In contrast to her sister Martha, who had been named Boston's debutante of the year, Ann–or Nan as John called her–was a graduate in mathematics from Bryn Mawr. She had also worked as an ambulance driver during World War I and had a reputation as a competent motor mechanic. The marriage proved to be most felicitous and the couple, by all accounts, were devoted to each other. By virtue of her mother's religion, Nan too, had been raised in the Catholic Church. Their marriage, on 3rd January, 1925, was one of the social events of the year, officiated as it was by none other than Cardinal William

O'Connell, a friend of Paul Thorndike's, and took place at the church of the Immaculate Conception, a prominent Boston church. It was rare for the cardinal to be thus employed, an indication of the influence and social prestige of the Thorndike family. Indeed, one of the few other marriages he had blessed before this was that of Joseph and Rose Kennedy in 1914.

A curious but telling anecdote is related of events preceding the ceremony that later had a significant influence on Rock's thinking. On the day prior to his wedding, he had performed a cesarean section, a contravention of church dogma. Confessing his "sin" to a local priest, he was told that he could not have absolution and hence the sacrament of marriage. Told of this, Cardinal O'Connell laughed the matter off, but later Rock mused on this schismatic interpretation of Catholic precepts.

His happy marriage to the 6-foot-tall Nan, one inch shorter than Rock, was blessed in quick succession with the birth of five children, the first in December 1925 and the last in February 1933. Their large, 13-room home became a chaotic scene of casually disciplined children, compounded by the family approbation for a number of canine pets. Despite the large home, Rock's indifferent attitude to the collection of medical fees kept the household finances in a constant precarious state. Whatever factors motivated John Rock, money was not one of them. Social status however, was one of those factors, and he became a member of some of Boston's more exclusive clubs open only to a few who were either members of the upper classes or high on the intellectual rungs of Boston society. This included the Tavern Club, a private club exclusively for men where his membership was once more facilitated by his brother-in-law Shermie and father-in-law Paul Thorndike, no mean accomplishment, given the suspicions with which Boston Catholics were regarded. It also helped that Nan was part of the Boston social register. Rock visited the club with some frequency, socializing with its prominent physicians and lawyers, later promoting the membership of Monsignor Francis Lally, a senior member of the church and first priest to be admitted to this austere group. In 1949, Rock was admitted to the even more exclusive Medical Exchange Club, limited to 12 members, of whom three were past Nobel Prize winners. Fortunately for John Rock, his older brother Charlie was gifted with considerable fiscal acumen and after the death of their father, Frank, was left as the trustee of his considerable fortune, estimated at $1.2 million in current dollars, which Charlie distributed to the family in time of need, but chiefly to John.

Before we review Rock's excursions into the field of birth control, it is well to take cognizance of the prevailing societal attitudes of the times toward the issue. As noted, the Catholic Church was fiercely opposed to contraception, as were indeed most of the Protestant churches. A break in this solid curtain of resistance came with the Lambeth Conference of 1930. This was a meeting in England of the bishops of the Anglican, or Episcopal, Church. It is held every 10 years at Lambeth Palace, the formal residence of the Archbishop of Canterbury, leader of the Church of England, the crown its titular head. There, for the first time, a vote by the majority of attendees in favor of limited approval of contraception, overcame a long tradition of calcified resistance, still reserving "strong condemnation of conception control from motives of selfishness, luxury or mere convenience." As if to condemn this faint liberal posture, later that same year (31st December, 1930), the Catholic Church under the direction of Pope Pius XI issued a papal encyclical, Casta Conubii, reaffirming that any artificial means of contraception was inherently wrong, opposed to nature, and equivalent to murder. In the following year, 1931, the redoubtable Margaret Sanger got up a petition to repeal the Massachusetts law opposing birth control. Here began Rock's apostasy. He, the sole Catholic among some 15 prominent Boston physicians, signed the petition. Rock had already begun to teach medical students what little that was then known of contraceptive measures, but signing the petition thrust his views into the glare of publicity, views regarded by his colleagues with almost universal disapproval, views that were anathema to his beloved church, views that flew in the face of the laws of Massachusetts, where not only was it illegal to use contraceptives but even to dispense information on the topic.

Rock continued his studies in infertility. Loretta McLaughlin, in her biography of Rock, quotes him on one clinical trial in which 80 infertile women were treated with estrogen and progesterone, the latter now available in quantity thanks to the work of Marker.[19] It was Rock's theory that infertility was due, at least in part, to underdevelopment of the uterus and that this might be corrected by hormonal treatment. In 1952 he embarked on this trial of "eighty frustrated but valiantly adventuresome patients to whom the experimental nature of the treatment and its unknown but probably harmless and only

---

19   The work and quote are so significant to the furtherance of contraception that it is repeated in Absell's biographical comments in "The Pill", in McLaughlin's biography of Rock, "The Pill, John Rock and the Church," and the biography of Marsh and Ronner. This study apparently was never published. In a search of Rock's papers at the Countyway Library of Harvard Medical School, there is a barely decipherable and heavily annotated report of this heterogeneous group of 80 infertile women. Rock made reference to this study in later publications. describing it as "in preparation." What was of greater significance in this study, other than the modest success in reversion of infertility, was of course, the realization that ovulation could be suppressed by the use of hormones. The quotation is taken from the text of Rock's presentation at the Laurentian Conference of 1956. The entire presentation was later published in 1957 under the title "Synthetic Progestins in the Normal Human Menstrual Cycle" (Recent Progress in Hormone Research 1957).

possibly helpful effects were carefully explained. Like us, they wanted to try it." It was well recognized from the clinical standpoint that the uterus enlarged very soon after conception in association with a rapid increase in circulating female hormones, specifically estrogen and progesterone but also a third, called chorionic gonadotropin derived from the placenta or after birth. Rock chose to use the former two. Chorionic gonadotropin was not utilized for several reasons: it lacked ready availability, required intramuscular administration and had some unpleasant side effects. Using the artificial estrogen diethylstilbestrol in ever-increasing dosages from 5 milligrams to 30 milligrams over a period of 11 weeks combined with progesterone in a dose of 50 milligrams, increasing to 300 milligrams, both given orally, he induced what he termed a "pseudo-pregnancy." Indeed, many of the women experienced the symptoms of early pregnancy, including breast tenderness and enlargement, nausea and above all, absence of menses, to the point that Rock had often to reassure his clientele and their husbands that, not only were they not pregnant but given the anti-ovulatory effect of the treatment, they could not become pregnant. Insofar as the goal of the experiment was the correction of infertility, the regime was moderately successful as 13 of the women conceived within four months, far more than would have occurred by chance alone.

As already noted, Rock's theory underlying this experiment was that some women had underdeveloped or infantile reproductive organs, that this was due to insufficient intrinsic hormones, and that this could be corrected by artificial substitution. However, it is likely that some of his patients in fact had undiagnosed endometriosis, a condition associated with infertility now treated by hormonal induction of amenorrhea (absent menses) for a duration of several months. It is frustrating that the details of his clinical trial were not

THE PEOPLE WHO MADE THE PILL

published in any scientific journal. Given by injection, progesterone is more effective than by the oral route, although the latter, given in the large doses that Rock ultimately used, was sufficiently effective.

It is recorded, without a precise date, that Rock and Pincus met fortuitously at a scientific meeting in 1952, where each is said to have learned of the work of the other, but almost certainly each must have had some prior passing acquaintance of the other's research through their publications. Pincus, successful in suppressing ovulation in rabbits and rats with progesterone, now saw that it was also possible in humans, although, in Rock's progesterone study, suppression of ovulation had not been his prime purpose. For Pincus, this must have been a revelation confirming what he must have suspected from his work on rabbits and rats, that is to say that suppression of ovulation by progesterone was efficacious in the human female.

At the suggestion of Pincus, Rock embarked on a second trial using progesterone alone. Selected for the trial were some 30 women with at least a two-year history of infertility in whom regular ovulation had been confirmed. Four became pregnant on cessation of progesterone treatment, but Pincus, on review of Rock's data, was critical of the laboratory evidence of ovulation suppression, noting that in some cases, this was uncertain. (One of the problems was that urinary pregnanediol, its presence a standard confirmation of ovulation, was also produced by the artificial administration of progesterone). Financial support for the studies became more and more important. It was around this time, in June of '53, that the historic meeting between Pincus, Margaret Sanger and Katharine McCormick took place, both women convinced that Pincus' research would produce an effective oral contraceptive. Not only did Pincus receive McCormick's immediate and substantial financial support,

196

but McCormick also gave financial support to Rock who, having reached the age of mandatory retirement from the Free Hospital when he became 65 on March 24, 1955, had been given a rundown building in which to pursue his work on infertility. When Katharine McCormick, aware of Rock's research, visited this facility, she was appalled at the cramped and wretched state of this building. In communication with Margaret Sanger she referred to it as "The Hovel." In the same year, she donated $100,000 towards its renovation. This was completed in 1957 and thenceforth became known as the Rock Reproductive Study Center.

Gregory Pincus, his laboratory research also supported by the Searle company, was aware of the progress in steroid research conducted by Djerassi, Colton and others, and now began to cast around for a compound that would not only suppress ovulation but would be consistently effective when given by mouth. Far from being a novice in steroid chemistry, Pincus had acquired considerable knowledge in the field. In his search for a more active progesterone, he was given, as we have noted in Chapter Five, access to several artificial progestins, among which were norethindrone, discovered by Djerassi, and norethynodrel, discovered later by Frank Colton. While he had access to both of these compounds, norethynodrel was readily available from the drug company Searle, along with company financial support, while norethindrone was mistakenly thought responsible for some masculinizing effects.

In a pair of articles published in the journal Science in 1956, Pincus and Chang first demonstrated the efficacy of oral progestins in suppressing ovulation in rodents. In the same issue Rock, Pincus and Garcia, in a study of infertile women, demonstrated suppression of ovulation in a group of 50 women using both norethindrone and norethynodrel in addition to a third, less-acceptable progestin.[20] Once more, these studies were performed ostensibly in the interest of correcting infertility, but it is clear from the study format that Rock and Pincus were primarily interested in the suppression of ovulation. While successful in this respect, they had to ask themselves many questions, such as which progestins were effective, in what dose, and with fewest side effects. Thus, the trial group of women was given dosages varying from 5 to 40 milligrams. Norethindrone and norethynodrel were each found to be equally, 100% effective in suppression of ovulation as measured by the absent urinary excretion of pregnanediol, the metabolite of progesterone; i.e. no pregnanediol, therefore no natural secretion of progesterone, and hence no ovulation. It was known that progesterone inhibited the pituitary hormones that stimulated the ovary to ovulate and produce natural progesterone, but they had to ask themselves if this was an exclusive inhibition. Might not progestins inhibit the production of other pituitary hormones, in particular adrenocorticotropin (ACTH), responsible for stimulating the adrenals in their production of cortisone? In this they were reassured by the absence of any measured decrease in urinary 17 keto-steroids, the metabolite of cortisone.

They also had to ask themselves the question, "What else might the progestins do?" While it was clear that they suppressed ovulation, would the ovaries recover normal function upon discontinuation of the progestins? In this they were reassured by the almost immediate return of evidence of ovulation in their study group as measured by the usual criteria of basal body temperature changes, ovulatory pattern of vaginal smears, and endometrial biopsies but, above all,

---

20   The same study was also published the following year in the American Journal of Obstetrics and Gynecology (vol 75 no.1), but in more detail and limited to the 40 women who took only either norethindrone or norethynodrel.

by the renewed levels of pregnanediol secretion. Further, out of 38 of these infertile patients treated exclusively with either norethindrone or norethynodrel, five became pregnant within five months of cessation of treatment, so that the potential problem of sterilization was put to rest. Additional support came from a small side study of seven women not included in the main study, but who were scheduled for abdominal surgery (hysterectomy with oophorectomy) for a variety of reasons. Rock treated these women with progestins for up to three months before surgery. Following surgery, their ovaries were examined both grossly and microscopically along with evaluation of endometrial (uterine) biopsies, which showed the ovaries to be quiescent with no evidence of ovulation, nor were the endometrial changes, while complex, consistent with ovulation. This microscopic work was performed by Dr. Angelika Tsacona, a Greek investigator working with Rock who, incidentally, received little formal recognition for her work. It is recorded that although there were then no formal standards of informed consent for this experimentation, Rock spent much time with his study patients explaining to them the risks, so far as he understood them. Even so, the potential for inducing cancerous changes in the reproductive organs was completely unknown and indeed, would not be known for many years.

What of these risks? It was one thing to suppress ovulation with drugs, but what if the side effects were intolerable or even life threatening? Fortunately, these proved to be benign and are well-recognized today in users of oral contraception. They included breast tenderness and enlargement, weight gain in a varying amount, nausea, fatigue and a variable effect on libido. (Most of these symptoms regress after one or two months on the pill.)

Meantime, Rock had enlisted as his assistants, the noted researcher, Dr. Ramon Celson-Garcia and Dr. Luigi Mastroianni, the former a Spanish American whose close ties to Puerto Rico were to prove significant and who later became professor and director of the Division of Human Reproduction at the University of Pennsylvania. Mastroianni was a young obstetrician from Yale, who also later became a professor and chairman of the Department of Obstetrics and Gynecology at University of Pennsylvania. Even before the studies were completed on Rock's sample of 50 women, Celson-Garcia, under Rock's supervision, conducted a contemporaneous study on 20 female medical students at the University of Puerto Rico with the more definitive intent of determining the efficacy of the progestins as contraceptives rather than as correctives of infertility. As noted in the previous chapter, this was legally permissible in Puerto Rico, which unlike the United States, and Massachusetts in particular, had no laws against contraception. However, when word of this leaked out to the predominantly Catholic faculty of the university, there was sufficient controversy that the program was curtailed. As previously noted in Chapter 8, there were other intrinsic problems with the study in that the subjects, well-educated women, were in no way similar to the poor, indigenous Puerto Rican women proposed for a later field study. To compound matters, the requirements of monthly collections of 48-hour urine specimens, daily temperature readings, and vaginal smears and monthly endometrial biopsies led to massive withdrawal of the candidates from the program.

One other concurrent study, this time completely unethical by contemporaneous standards, took place at the Worcester State Hospital, a facility for the treatment of mental illness. The institution had long been supported by Katharine McCormick, her interest in mental illness stimulated by the insanity of Stanley McCormick, her long-incarcerated husband. She had, as far back as 1927, instituted and financially supported its Neuroendocrine Research Foundation. Thus, the administration had little difficulty and much incentive in agreeing to the experiment on seven women and eight men, all of whom were psychotics. There was some rationale in protecting the women from pregnancy, which occurred from time to time despite institutional protection from this risk. But it was quite impossible to engage the cooperation of the men in production of specimens of semen. Most of the men under treatment displayed evidence of feminization, which was reversible. Despite these distractions, there was no doubt from Rock's 50-woman study that the progestins norethindrone and norethynodrel were effective contraceptives with seemingly only benign and temporary side effects.

By all reports, Pincus, Sanger and McCormick were ecstatic in their response to these trials, while Rock remained only cautiously optimistic, acutely aware of the legal, ethical and religious opposition to their work. It is reported that he was unhappy that the first reports of the work using progestins alone were delivered by Pincus at the meeting of the fifth conference of the International Planned Parenthood League, held in Tokyo in October 1955. At that time, the studies had not been published and, consequently, not subjected to professional scrutiny. Significantly, Rock refused to attend the conference. His anticipation of the coming controversial storm over his work proved remarkably prescient, but was not provoked by Pincus' presentation at the conference. Although the results of the study, looked at objectively, were quite breathtaking, they were greeted with a collective yawn, disinterest and lack of curiosity.

Here, at the conference was proposed long-term medication of otherwise healthy women, not for any disease but simply to defer or avoid pregnancy, medication whose long-term side effects were not only unknown but also unknowable and would be unknowable for many years. However, in this instance, Rock need scarcely have worried. As noted, Pincus' presentation was received with little attention, even skepticism, its potential little realized, if at all. Nevertheless, Rock was greatly irritated.

The next year, 1956, was a watershed year. This was when Pincus published his rat studies in the journal Science, showing the anti-ovulatory effect of the progestins. In the same issue, Rock published his study of the 50 women treated with progestins. The choice of the journal Science was probably predicated on Pincus' membership in the American Association for the Advancement of Science (AAAS) but it seemed a peculiar choice for Rock, for the journal Science, while of great general appeal to the scientific community, would reach few obstetricians/gynecologists and perhaps was a reflection of Rock's reticence in making his revelations more widely known. The great epiphany came at the Laurentian Conference held in early 1956. The annual Laurentian conferences were sponsored by AAAS and were held at Mont Tremblant in the mountains of Quebec beginning in 1944. It attracted attendees whose main interest was in endocrinology rather than the wider field of medicine.

At the conference, Rock, after a brief review of his earlier studies, all ostensibly aimed at correcting infertility, gave a long and detailed presentation on the results of his trial on the use of progestins in his group of 50 infertile women in whom ovulation had been confirmed and who, prior to medication, had regular menses. Thirty three of these 50 had never been pregnant; 13 had borne at least one child, and the remaining four had conceived but miscarried. Of these 50, 40 were treated either with norethindrone or norethynodrel. Of the

10 remaining women who were treated with a third progestin, the evidence for suppression of ovulation was incomplete and less robust.

In his presentation, Rock carefully reviewed the standard criteria for proof of ovulation and of their absence during treatment with progestins, considering as he did so possible alternative explanations for their absence. These criteria, already described, were absence of temperature elevation in mid-cycle, failure of changes in vaginal smears consistent with ovulation, unusual appearance of the endometrial lining inconsistent with ovulation, and above all, low secretion of urinary pregnanediol. To bolster his theory, he also described his seven surgical cases pretreated with norethindrone wherein there was no evidence of ovulation. The only objective side effect was a slight lengthening of the menstrual cycle with delayed bleeding. All 50 women resumed ovulatory cycles on termination of the medication and none conceived during treatment. However, seven out of 38 treated with either norethindrone or norethynodrel became pregnant within five months of treatment cessation which, taken together with resumption of normal menses, was reassuring that there were no long-term adverse side effects. Of course, Rock presented this as a small but probably significant effect on infertility of the progestins.

His presentation evoked much discussion among the attendees including the suggestion, later confirmed, that some of the investigators were using progestins contaminated with an estrogen of some potency. This was later confirmed, but removal of the identified estrogen, mestranol, reduced the potency of the contraceptive effect.

The most enlightened comment came from Dr. David Greenblatt, later a pioneer in the use of norgestrel, a latter-day progestin. He is quoted as saying, "One fact which stood out in this study is that Dr. Rock has *unwittingly* given us an excellent oral contraceptive which may be employed with little untoward effect. It appears that these progesterone-like substances are capable of inhibiting ovulation if the proper schedule is employed."

Whether or not Rock smiled at this observation, is not recorded!

The first application for use as a contraceptive was filed on 29th October, 1959. It was not rebuffed, but the FDA used a delaying tactic: If it could not, or did not come to a decision within 90 days, the applicant could be notified that the filing would be delayed for six months. The FDA used this tactic twice. Incredibly, it transpired that the FDA was using a part-time reviewer fresh out of residency training in obstetrics and gynecology named Pasquale DeFelice, a mere 35 years old at the time. Residency training at that time was a mandatory three years after graduation from medical school and a year of internship. Nor was he board certified, the ultimate imprimatur of the specialist obtained only after passage of rigorous board examinations. Professionally, one could compare DeFelice as a midget dealing in his field with the giant of John Rock. The story, as told by I.C. Winter, is a bureaucratic aphorism.

Besides his woeful inexperience, and although he denied it, DeFelice was almost certainly the prisoner of orthodox Catholic precepts on the issue of contraception. He was educated not only at Fordham University, a repository of Jesuit philosophy, but had his medical education at Georgetown, a respected but equally Catholic-oriented institution, once more of Jesuit origination. If any doubt should be imputed to the influence of his educational antecedents, it should be noted that later in life he fathered 10 children.

At first, DeFelice delayed approval on the irrational grounds that proof was lacking that it in fact did work, using the analogy that "someone could submit an application for sterile water in the treatment of arthritis and if you couldn't prove that it didn't work – rather than it did – it would be approved." His logic was erroneous on two grounds. First, the FDA did require proof that a drug was effective, and second, as DeFelice conceded, the testing and documentation of the pill for side effects far exceeded that of any prior drug application. Of course, it was a completely novel concept that a woman would take a daily pill, not for a disease but to prevent pregnancy and DeFelice, as even he admitted, had one eye cast over his shoulder with regard to job security.

I.C. Winter, as the representative of the Searle company, the formal applicant, finally asked for a hearing and so, accompanied by the company's medical director, Dr. J. William Crosson, and, at their invitation, Dr. Rock, they met with DeFelice. By all accounts the meeting took place in late December of 1959 on an extremely cold day. The building where they were to meet the FDA representative was a wooden temporary building constructed as a barracks during World War II. Rock, now close to 70 years old, and his two companions were kept waiting and standing for an hour and a half in an unheated entrance way pending the arrival of DeFelice, whose youth startled and confounded them. This was the individual charged with the climactic decision of approval, a person who had kept them waiting without excuse, probably with the intention of discouraging them. But it was Rock who carried the discussion.

DeFelice raised a number of objections. He was critical of the paucity, to him, of the studies, although they were considerable and had been assiduously reviewed by Rock and Celson Garcia, each having personally checked the record of every patient. In an affront to Rock's experience DeFelice raised the issue of carcinogenicity, but Rock, having seen that the contraceptive pill acted by causing a pseudo-pregnancy and aware from his observations over a long professional career that fertile women were less prone to cancer, angrily countered, noting DeFelice's limited experience. Finally, DeFelice raised the moral issue, asserting that the Catholic Church would never approve, which led Rock to accuse him of "selling my church short." In the end, DeFelice tried to assuage the group by promising to send the data to outside consultants and referees. Rock, who throughout the discussion referred to DeFelice as "young man," furious at this inept youth, grasped him by the lapels, and told him that he, DeFelice, would decide right now!

Later reviewing the interview, Rock was quoted as saying, "In came a nondescript 30-year-old from Washington. Can you imagine, the FDA gave *him* the job of deciding? I was furious." Later, DeFelice had quite a different take on the interview, lauding Rock as a great professional figure. He accused the Searle representatives of asking for immediate approval of a reduction in the dosage of Enovid from 10 milligrams to 5 milligrams or even as low as 2.5, accusing them of being motivated by profit, because the larger dose was more expensive to produce. He was able to introduce a minor impediment to approval by insisting that studies be performed to ensure that the medication would not cause blood clotting, on the theory that pregnant women were more prone to this complication. On April 22nd, 1960, approval was mailed on condition of some minor labeling changes. This done, the official release became effective on the historic date of 11th May, 1960.

CHAPTER TEN

Epilogue

"And what good came of it all at last?" quoth little Peterkin.
"Why, that I cannot say," said he, "but 'twas a famous victory."

With the 1960 Food and Drug Administration approval of the pill for contraception, the primary goals of Sanger, Pincus, McCormick and Rock in providing safe, effective reversible contraception remote from the sex act itself were finally met with far-reaching and, to some extent, unpredictable consequences. The mere availability led to widespread public discussion of the whole field of contraception. This topic, hitherto hardly fit for polite conversation, was now increasingly introduced into the arena of public debate and comment. It opened up avenues for the advent of alternative methods of contraception, their prospective use now more or less free of the philosophic and religious opposition that they had historically faced. Foams, condoms, diaphragms, jellies, contraceptive pills and intrauterine devices all became matters of open discussion as to costs, advantages, side effects and pregnancy rates, and with it, a widening acceptance of sterilization for both males and females.

For example, as a newcomer to our local hospital in the late '60s I proposed liberalizing our hospital rules regarding sterilization.

At that time, we had a three-man (and I do mean man) sterilization committee that would agree to the procedure in certain cases, and only such cases, where pregnancy represented a significant health hazard. Local physicians who were opposed to liberalization informed me that elective sterilization was illegal. Thus I, as an immigrant to the U.S., accepted this until informed by a more enlightened colleague that such legal proscriptions were nonexistent. By way of further investigation, I took it upon myself to write to the legal advisors of our state medical society seeking an opinion. Their response, while indicating that there was nothing illegal pertaining to sterilization, declared that such an operation might later be deemed as having no clinical indication and thus could be interpreted as grounds for charges of assault with litigious consequences! Seeking the policies of other hospitals located in our state, I received the most cautious and restrained replies indicating restrictive attitudes to the procedure. However, my persistence resulted in a change of our hospital by-laws permitting the elective performance of female sterilization. The reader will be astonished to learn that permission would be granted only to women who met the following criteria:

- Age 25 with five children.

- Age 30 with four children.

- Age 35 with 3 children.

Application had to be made in writing to the hospital's Committee on Sterilization and Abortion and had to be signed by both the woman and her husband! This was in the early '70s. Similar strictures were placed on male sterilization, but it soon became evident that vasectomies could easily be performed in a physician's office under local anesthesia without the need for hospitalization or any application for permission. Of course, sterilization has been totally liberalized since then and is now simply an elective procedure based solely on the patient's discretion and a willing physician. Indeed, it is the most popular method of contraception among couples over 30 years of age, although the ratio of female to male is 2:1.

Learned epidemiologic reviews of each method of contraception were published in a variety of medical journals. Pregnancy rates and side effects were widely documented. Studies on the effectiveness of the oral contraceptive pill showed a pregnancy rate of .03% in consistent users of the medication as distinct from those who either forgot one or more pills, had been given improper instruction in their use, or who deliberately discontinued them. Overall, the pregnancy rate varied from 2%-8%. International approval swiftly followed U.S. approval by the FDA. Britain, Canada, Australia and Germany gave approval in the following year and France, where the decision was delayed by necessary changes in the law, followed in 1967.

Even in the United States, despite governmental approval, legal barriers persisted in some states until finally removed by the 1965 watershed decision of the United States Supreme Court in Griswold v. Connecticut. Incredible though it may seem to the modern reader, until this landmark decision of the Supreme Court, Connecticut still had laws that prohibited contraception. These, while scarcely enforced, had already been tested unsuccessfully before the Supreme Court, but to test the law once more, Estelle Griswold, executive director of the Planned Parenthood League of Connecticut, and Lee Buxton, a professor at Yale School of Medicine, opened a birth control clinic in New Haven with the express intention of testing the law. They were shortly arrested, tried, convicted and fined $100 each. Their convictions were upheld by an Appellate Court and later the Supreme Court of Connecticut, before their successful appeal to the United States Supreme Court, where the decisions of the lower courts were overturned based on the argument of "right to marital privacy." Although the latter is not specifically mentioned in the Constitution, the court based its decision largely on the argument that privacy was protected by the Due-Process Clause of the 14th Amendment. However, this decision protected marital couples only. Subsequently, in the 1972 decision of Eisenstadt v. Baird, protection was extended to non-married couples based on the Equal Protection Clause of the 14th Amendment.

Thus the legal barriers limiting contraceptive advice exclusively to married couples were breached, changing traditional sexual mores forever. For example, this author well remembers what then seemed to him an excruciating dilemma he faced when, in the mid 1960s, the young, unmarried daughter of one of his colleagues applied to him for a prescription for the pill. Reluctantly agreeing, he later mentioned to his colleague that he had given a prescription to an anonymous unmarried girl asking him for his philosophy, whereupon his colleague agreed with the (my) decision, thus salving this author's conscience. Nowadays, such conservatism in most quarters would provoke only a smile. A curious exception to the widespread international acceptance took place in Japan, where the pill was not approved until 1999. Abortion in Japan was, and is, legal. It is widely accepted there, so that population growth, a major concern, has been controlled. The delay in approval was due, paradoxically to the resistance of the Japanese Medical Association, which used the argument that the wide use of condoms prevented sexually transmitted diseases. Some justification for this was later provided by the low incidence of AIDS in Japanese society, but one is led to suspect that much of the resistance was due to the financial returns from provision of medical abortions.

Side effects of the pill became an issue in particular when it became apparent that women who used it were prone to pulmonary embolus, a sometimes-fatal disease. Pulmonary embolus is caused by blood clots formed in the deep veins of the legs which, when released into the bloodstream, travel directly to the pulmonary circulation and block blood flow to the lungs, causing chest pain, shortness of breath, and even death. There is little doubt that this is indeed a risk factor, but since it was identified, the estrogen and progestin content of the pill, considered to be causative, have been dramatically reduced. In addition, it has become clear that certain women are more prone to this serious complication such as those who are obese, are smokers, or are older than 35 years, so that requests from women under these circumstances are generally declined. Something that is often lost in the safety argument is that pregnancy itself carries a variety of risk factors, including blood clotting and pulmonary embolus. Thus, there is still today a moderate but significant mortality from pregnancy (6/10,000), a factor usually overlooked in the debates over contraception and abortion. There are of course, additional minor side effects, such as breast tenderness and nausea, that usual regress after the first month or two of usage. Intermenstrual bleeding, or spotting, although harmless, is common, often difficult to control, and the bane of the gynecologist.

While the risk of cancer has often been invoked and at first was difficult to refute due to the longtime follow-up necessary to determine risk, it is now apparent that the risk of cancer of the reproductive organs is reduced among women taking the pill. The best example is of ovarian cancer, a highly lethal form of malignancy, which not only is reduced in users of oral contraception, but also is reduced in proportion to length of usage. Likewise, cancer of the endometrium, or uterine lining, has a lower incidence in pill users.

Birth Rates, Fertility, Population Growth, and the Economic Effects on Women

Sanger's goals were threefold. Primarily and essentially, she wanted to offer women a safe alternative to unwanted, multiple child-bearing, and in this she was overwhelmingly successful. Her other goal was to control the dramatic growth in world population. In this she was quite unsuccessful, for it will be seen that, as is generally known, during the past 100 years or so, the world population has not only burgeoned dramatically but also is predicted to continue to do so. And not only has population increased, but so also has the rate of increase.

Appended are three graphs demonstrating the changes in birth rate and fertility rate and total births in the U.S. following the release of the oral contraceptive in 1957.

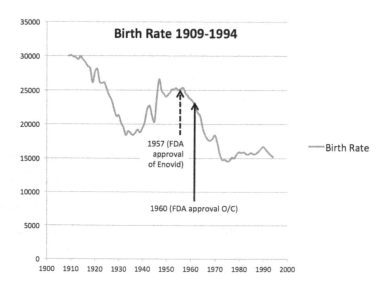

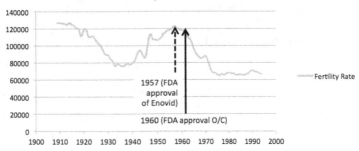

Fertility Rate 1909-1994

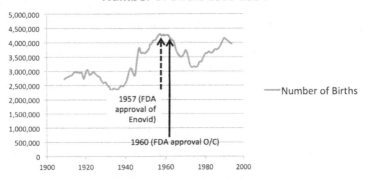

Number of Births 1909-1994

The reader should be aware of some significant differences between certain birth statistics. Total number of births, as expected, generally will rise with population increase, which in the U.S. has been constantly rising, for obviously the more people there are, the greater the likelihood of a rise in the number of births. But certain factors will skew this figure. Clearly an aging population will not be as potentially productive as a younger one for the obvious reason that older women are no longer fertile. What is of much more significance in childbirth statistics is the fertility rate, which is the number of children born per 1,000 women ages 15 to 44, and in this we see a precipitous and sustained decline beginning with the release in 1957 of the pill for menstrual disorders, not yet approved for contraception, but quickly recognized by women as an effective method of birth control.

This should not be concluded as entirely cause and effect, for no doubt there are other social factors involved such as increased employment and educational opportunities for women and the reduction in the burden of common household chores, relieved in part by modern kitchen and laundry appliances. Indeed, hitherto the lowest birth rates per 1,000 population in the U.S. were recorded at the depths of the Depression of the 1930s when methods of contraception were either primitive or unknown. The all-time low was recently recorded for 2010, when, although there were 4,136,000 births, the birth rate was 13.5 per 1,000, once more a reflection of difficult economic times due to a prolonged recession.

To reiterate, the fertility rate is not to be confused with the birth rate (second graph from top), which also has decreased. As a population ages, as has happened in the United States, the proportion of women of childbearing age decreases and as a consequence birth rate per 1,000 drops, regardless of the availability of contraception. As can also be seen from the top graph, despite the steady growth in the population of the United States, the total number of births has risen only moderately over the past 30 years and is now barely level with the peak year of 1961 (4,268,326 births). When one compares the birth rates and fertility rates with, say, the early 20th century—which were, from 1909 until 1929, respectively 123-107 (fertility rate or number of children born to women between 15 and 44) and 30-26 (birth rate or number of births per 1,000 population) — it will be seen further that there has been a dramatic change, but none so dramatic as the years following the introduction of the pill.

Clearly there are other factors at work. Changes from an agricultural society to an industrial one require fewer children to work the land so that children, instead of being potential farmhands, become economic liabilities. Other economic factors influence these statistics, as witnessed by the decline in fertility and birth rates synchronous with the Great Depression of the 1930s. One can only speculate on the causes at that time, but certainly the economic constrictions of the Great Depression probably resulted in delayed marriage and greater use of whatever unsophisticated methods of contraception were available, i.e. condoms and withdrawal.

Figure 1
Student Matriculations by Gender 1858/59 – 1993/94

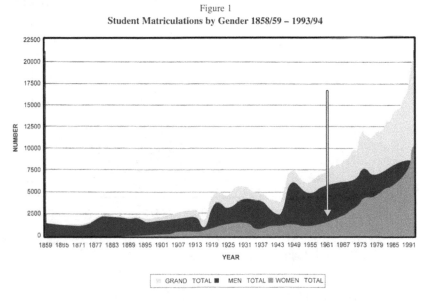

Arrowhead shows 1961 approval of oral contraceptives in U.K.

Above is a graph of admissions (defined by "matriculation") by sex to the University of Glasgow in the U.K. dating from 1859. I have chosen my alma mater for reasons of simplicity of access to data. Such data are difficult to obtain from American colleges and are skewed by the large number of colleges that, until relatively recently, were open only to women, such as Vassar, Wellesley, etc. The reader will notice the rise in the proportion of women undergraduates beginning in the late '50s, rising rapidly in the '60s until, by the early '90s, women made up the larger proportion by sex, again concurrent with the approval of the oral contraceptive in the U.K. in 1961. Once more, this should be interpreted with caution, for surely other social factors were at work, but it is an interesting juxtaposition that invites speculation.

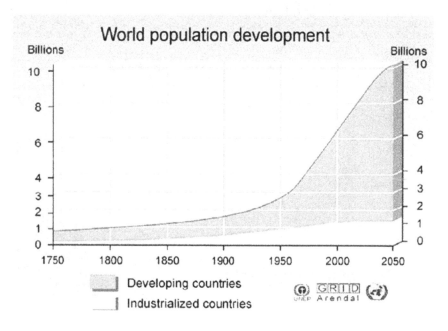

Sanger's second goal in her search for an effective contraceptive was her concern over the rapid growth in world population and the Malthusian concern that population would outgrow food supply. Not only has there been no overall effect on world population reduction but, on the contrary, world population has risen dramatically at an ever-increasing rate, more than trebling in a mere 100 years between 1900 and 2000. With the green revolution and improvements in plant genetics, the limitations on food supply have not occurred and indeed, the overall nutrition of the human populace has greatly improved. Nevertheless, such a rate of population growth cannot be sustained forever. Apart from nutritional considerations, there is increasing evidence that population pressures are causing deterioration in the world environment, with loss or threatened loss of species through reduction of habitat from human encroachment. A primary example is the increase in atmospheric concentration of carbon dioxide due to the consumption of fossil fuels, which, in turn, is thought by many to be responsible for some degree of global warming. Whether the theory is accurate or not, its basis is certainly attributable to population growth. Some slight solace might be taken in that the rate of population increase has recently slowed.

Despite the worldwide dramatic increase in population, the more industrialized societies show evidence of population decline, a concern for those nativists who place a premium on, and would like to preserve, western culture, religion and values, for only by immigration from less-developed countries can their populations be sustained. The fact of their higher standards of living makes them attractive to people from relatively impoverished areas of the world whose language, educational background and values are often at variance.

Eugenics

Sanger's third goal was in the field of eugenics, aimed at the reduction of mental retardation and birth defects by limiting the reproduction of the "unfit." Simple observation suggested that the children of bright, intelligent people seemed more likely to be bright and intelligent themselves, whereas the converse also seemed true, i.e. the children of the mentally slow were more likely to be similarly afflicted. For the most part, these theories, consonant with Sanger's times, ignored the significance of environmental factors and failed to take cognizance of the better educational opportunities the affluent provided to their offspring. The eugenic theories of Sanger's time have largely been looked at askance, scientific support lacking. In addition, the entire concept was widely discredited by the uninformed and biased policies of the Nazi regime in Germany during the '30s and '40s where even ethnic groups, Jews primarily but also the Slavic peoples, were viewed as untermenschen, or subhuman. The ethical controversy persists, however. It is now possible in some instances to predetermine the fetal potential not only for mental retardation, but also for certain physical illnesses, by evaluation of the genetic potential of the parents or diagnosis of abnormal fetuses in utero. Down's syndrome is the classic example. Screening tests for it during pregnancy are now widely available, but the decision on the fate of the fetus ultimately is that of the mother-to-be. It is also possible to screen parents for their genetic potential for Huntingdon's chorea, Tay-Sachs disease, sickle cell anemia, and cystic fibrosis. Huntingdon's chorea is a devastating form of inherited mental illness and dementia that does not manifest itself until well into adulthood; Tay-Sachs disease is generally limited to the children of parents of Jewish ancestry, and leads to death in early infancy; sickle cell disease is generally confined to black people and is manifested by painful hemolytic crises that are sometimes lethal. Life expectancy is curtailed; cystic fibrosis is a disease that chronically disables the child due to respiratory and digestive problems, so that life expectancy is limited to little beyond early adulthood. Whether to prevent or abort such pregnancies is at least arguable. The ethical dilemma becomes more formidable in the determination of minor defects. For example, Turner's syndrome produces a child who is phenotypically female, but is missing one of the two X chromosomes of the normal woman, so-called X0 in genetic terms. Superficially, such children would pass as normal or nearly so. Although they are seldom of more than average intelligence, they are of short stature, fail to develop secondary sexual characteristics, and are infertile. Particularly abhorrent is the termination of pregnancy where ultra sound demonstrates the presence of a female fetus. This approach is not unusual in some countries, particularly in Asia, where there is a premium on male offspring.

And what of the other side of the coin? It is now possible for a woman to select the father of her child from a variety of sperm and/or egg donors. While restricted, in general, to couples with irremediable infertility, it has been used for production of families for single women or homosexual females. Donors chosen are usually well-educated males and most often of Caucasian ancestry, a reflection of the continuing bias against people with darker skins.

Current Views

While the religious fervor that stirred opposition to contraception has largely receded, it is by no means dormant. One has only to look at some restrictive governmental policies for an awareness of bias toward contraception, an example being the limitations of American aid to African countries that have liberal approaches to abortion. Under the recent administration of George W. Bush, the American government program PEPFAR (President's Emergency Plan for Relief of AIDS) provided funds in the billions of dollars with the strict proviso that no monies were to be used for contraception or counseling on birth control. A small country like Uganda—roughly the size of Nebraska with a population expected to triple to 96 million over the next 40 years and an average birth rate of 6.7 children per woman, one of the highest in the world—thus has difficulty in controlling its burgeoning growth. Of course the problem is compounded by African tribal traditions, taboos, patriarchal customs, and the economic difficulties of providing effective public health systems. In addition, the Roman Catholic Church is the largest Ugandan Christian denomination and remains opposed to contraception, having fought to retain the Bush limitations.

Other examples of religious opposition abound. As recently as 2005 the Food and Drug Administration, under the influence of the religious right, declined approval of marketing the "morning-after pill" without a prescription.[21] The morning-after pill was promoted as a method of preventing conception where unprotected intercourse had taken place within the past 72 hours. Approved, but by prescription only, as early as 1999, its effectiveness was severely limited by the obvious difficulty of quickly receiving a prescription from an available and willing physician and having it filled in a reasonable amount of time at a pharmacy that held the medication in stock, thus rendering this approval largely impractical. Further, the efficacy of this so-called Plan B as it became known, declines steadily as the time interval extends from the origin of the sex act to ingestion of the medication. Therefore, the risk of pregnancy increases from an estimated .4% if initiated within 24 hours, to 2.7% if initiated between 48 and 72 hours. The difficulties are further compounded by the likelihood that sexual activity took place over the weekend when resources are less accessible.

Responding to a request from the manufacturer that the medication be made available without prescription, the FDA arranged

21   New England Journal of Medicine; September, 22 2005: "A Sad Day for Science at the FDA"

a meeting of experts both in the fields of obstetrics and gynecology and in over-the-counter drug availability, who voted 23 to 4 for approval. The dissenters admitted that their opposition had no basis in concern for side effects or safety, which should have been the sole concerns of the FDA. The professional staff of the FDA supported this decision for approval. Nevertheless, the proposal was rejected by the management, concerned that availability would increase the frequency of sexual behavior in young adults despite the fact that this was merely conjectural and unsupported by evidence. Later the agency was quite unable to provide a scintilla of evidence to back this contention. Safety had already been approved in a December 2003 meeting by a vote of 28 to 0. Nevertheless, in a 2004 decision, it was decided to limit over-the-counter purchase to women 16 and older, while others would require a prescription, a unique duality for any drug. As pointed out in the New England Journal article, many over-the-counter drugs can, in inappropriate dosages, be quite hazardous to health and even lethal. Acetaminophen (sold as Tylenol and other brand names) is unrestricted for purchase by young people, and its over-ingestion leads annually to more than 56,000 emergency room visits, 26,000 hospital admissions, and more than 450 deaths. Citing recent studies, the article further refuted the arguments that provision of the morning-after pill led to promiscuity, greater incidence of sexually transmitted diseases, and under-utilization of more effective contraceptive measures. Enforcement of the prescription requirement would have resulted in the humiliation of the purchaser, who would have to be "carded," thus revealing to the pharmacy clerk, be it male or female, that she had had unprotected intercourse within the past 24 hours.

In protest of these unscientific decisions, Dr. Susan Wood, professor of medicine and pharmacology at Vanderbilt School of Medicine, member of the FDA Advisory Committee on Non-prescription Drugs, and director of the agency's Office of Women's Health, submitted her resignation. At the time of writing, the morning-after pill still requires a prescription for those under 17. However, studies have shown that the rates of abortion are unchanged between users of Plan B and non-users.

Abortion

Abortion is a medical term defined as the termination of a pregnancy before the stage of viability. It can be, and often is, spontaneous, so in fact, upward of 15% of pregnancies end in abortion or, to use the lay term, "miscarriage." Throughout this section, the term abortion will be used to describe the intentional termination of pregnancy–so-called induced abortion.

Widely accepted as a means of birth control, particularly in Russia and until recently the principle method in Japan, the role of induced abortion remains one of fiery controversy despite its legalization in America in the epic Supreme Court decision of Roe v. Wade (22nd January, 1973). It will come as a surprise to most readers that, until the end of the 18th century, there was no law prohibiting early abortion for the simple reason that pregnancy could not be confirmed until "quickening," which is not apparent until at least 16 weeks of gestation. Even this depended on the parity of the mother, for women who have never borne a child will usually not recognize fetal movement until 18 weeks. Thus early pregnancy could be terminated by pleading ignorance of the nature of missed menses, a claim that, although disingenuous in many cases, provided legal cover. It is clear from the adverts of the time, couched in euphemistic terms such as "guarantees of success in all female complaints," that knowledge of abortion services was pervasive and that they were widely sought. That they were effectual is a different matter. For all the varied concoctions, purgatives, botanicals, extracts of juniper berries (savin), leaves of ivy or willow, few if any would stand up to modern scientific appraisal, and some were downright lethal.[22] Indeed, inasmuch as savin, derived from the commonplace juniper bush, was the preferred drug because of its ready availability and low cost, deaths in the 19th century from overdosage of this drug were not uncommon.

An alternative to these drugs, or abortifacients, was instrumental intercession. It was widely known and even taught in medical schools that dilatation of the cervix, or mouth of the womb, with or without rupture of the membranes (bag of waters) would induce abortion. Not that this was without hazard. In an era preceding antiseptic surgery, infection, with or without mortal consequences, must have been frequent. Further, at a time preceding any type of anesthesia, or even before the invention of a vaginal speculum that would provide adequate visualization, the procedure must have been, to say the least, uncomfortable and prone to inaccurate manipulation.

---

22   John Riddle, in his book "Contraception and Abortion from the Ancient World to the Renaissance," gives an erudite and inclusive account of the varied pharmacological interventions of Greek, Roman and Arabic physicians recommended for both contraception and abortion and claiming at least moderate effectiveness. He alleges that knowledge of such methods has been lost since the advent of formal medical education beginning in the 15th century and that such education was restricted to males. However, while some efficacy has been demonstrated in laboratory animals, few of these methods have been subjected to formal scientific evaluation or reported in the more conventional medical publications.

As contraceptives, they were prescribed either just before or just after the onset of menses in the mistaken belief that these were the peak fertile periods of the human female. This has since been completely controverted by the knowledge that ovulation takes place in midcycle.

Before dealing with the oncoming legal changes of the 19th century, it should be conceded that there were longstanding ethical concerns on the topic of induced abortion, the most well-known being the section of the Hippocratic Oath which, paraphrased, reads, "I will not give a woman an abortive remedy." In Chaucer's "Parson's Tale," the narrator inveighs against disturbance of the conception of a child. There are other not-infrequent proscriptions in Western literature opposing abortion, but the term was ill-defined and it is probable that these interdictions were related to pregnancies in which quickening had manifested itself.

In the United States, the only legal restriction on abortion was derived from English common law, enforceable only after quickening and rarely pursued by the courts. In the beliefs of the time, until quickening took place, the fetus was not considered a living entity. Aside from any moral argument, in the absence of any objective test of pregnancy, proof of gestation was lacking. It would be naive to suppose that any sexually active woman of childbearing age would not have reason to recognize her status after missing a period or two, for besides the obvious symptom of amenorrhea, she would also notice breast enlargement and tenderness, nausea and possibly vomiting, urinary frequency, and that fatigue peculiar to the first three months of gestation. Further, the uterus enlarges, which is detectable by pelvic examination, and becomes palpable abdominally as early as 12 weeks.

In the convenient rationalization of the times, the menses were "obstructed" and the obstruction might be relieved by medication or instrumental interference. For, if no one knew for certain of the woman's condition, there could hardly be any reproach for dealing with a minor female problem. Moreover, the cause of obstruction could be assigned to serious, if undefined, threats to the woman's health.

It is true that the British Parliament in 1803 passed more restrictive laws, known as the Ellenborough Laws after their chief proponent, Lord Ellenborough, making abortion illegal even before quickening. Although aware of this change in British forensics, American legislatures, with a degree of uniformity amounting to unanimity, chose to ignore the British statutes. For example, in a trial before the Supreme Court of Massachusetts in 1812, plaintiff Isaiah Bangs, accused of attempting abortion by providing an abortifacient, was exonerated on the grounds that quickening had not taken place. The case established a precedent that was followed by the remaining states for the next 40 years or so. Succinctly, this can be expressed by the dictum, "No quickening, ergo, no pregnancy."

Data on the frequency, safety and demographics of early- to mid-19-century abortions are, at best, speculative, but it would seem, in the absence of multiple reportings of post-abortion deaths, that it was relatively safe. There can be little doubt that abortion was resorted to as a solution for unwanted pregnancy. However, the consensus was that it was used primarily by young, unwed women for whom there was some societal sympathy, relieving them, as it did, of the shame of illegitimacy. It seems that at that time it was an uncommon resort of the married woman.

As the 19th century progressed, all this began to change. Beginning around the 1840s until the 1870s, abortion became commercialized. Increasingly, in response to the revenue derived therefrom, the press carried multiple advertisements for abortion services, albeit couched in the most recondite terms. Although, beginning in 1821 with a law passed by the Connecticut legislature,[23] state statutes were passed dealing specifically with abortion, these were largely unenforceable due, once more, to the concept of quickening as the only confirmatory evidence of pregnancy.

In the decade from 1840 to 1850, abortion became commonplace, widely used not only for relief from the burdens of pregnancy, illegitimate or otherwise, but increasingly as a method of contraception. The change effected several consequences, each of which disturbed the contemporary social fabric. There was a steady fall in the birth rate, which in and of itself was a concern for the young republic. But worse, in the eyes of nativists and eugenecists, the solicitors of abortion services were no longer poor single women but mostly married, white, Protestant women of the middle and upper classes, women who constituted the original Anglo Saxon establishment. One commentator was provoked into speculating that in 50 years, a white, fair-haired, blue-eyed individual would become a rarity!

A second reaction took place in the medical profession. In the absence of formal licensing, the profession was divided arbitrarily into

23   Passed by the Connecticut legislature in 1821. it considered the profoundly deleterious effects of some remedies advocated by abortionists, chiefly by physicians and apothecaries, which were becoming increasingly recognized. The law made it illegal to administer any toxic substance harmful to a pregnant woman's health or life. In this it should be noted that the outcome to the fetus was secondary, the prime concern being preservation of the life and health of the mother. It was in effect, a poison-control measure. Abortion by instrumentation was unaffected. It is conjectured that passage of this law was based on the passage in Great Britain in 1803 of the so-called Ellenborough Laws, which made abortion after quickening, a capital offense, but in addition made it illegal prior to quickening and punishable by transportation. While the Connecticut law limited itself to poisoning and, at that, only after quickening, and held the woman blameless, the British law was much more comprehensive, exposing criminal risk to any abortion attempt and even holding the woman in legal jeopardy.

two groups, the regulars and the irregulars. The regulars consisted for the most part of physicians who had had at least some formal education. The irregulars were simply individuals who hung out their shingles, as it were, and proceeded to practice medicine. The latter, as abortionists, were able to sequester to themselves the better-paying female patients, who, in turn, tended to return for further care with or without their families. Thus the profession was faced with a significant economic problem epitomized by the enormous financial success of the famous, or notorious, abortionist Madam Restell, with whom we have dealt in Chapter One.

The press, in a perverse counter to their main revenue source, began to publish lurid accounts of women fatally injured in the abortion process. When Madame Restell was arrested for the second time in 1845, her court case was closely followed by the mainstream newspapers. However, as advertising revenue increased, the press published fewer and fewer such articles beginning in the '50s.

In 1847, in defense of the economic interests of the profession against nonqualified practitioners, the "regulars" formed the American Medical Association and, following that, established the state medical societies. In 1857, one of its more active members, Horatio Robinson Storer, embarked on a long crusade against abortion, enlisting the help of not only his medical colleagues but also enrolling the help of reluctant church leaders. The actions of physicians were primarily based on the moral issue of extinguishing fetal life, for it was becoming more apparent to the profession that fetal life preceded quickening. Less spoken of in their arguments was the inherent nativism and prejudicial attitudes of the physicians of the time, who were almost exclusively white, Protestant and male. A third reason was the opposition to the changing role of women in society. Women were becoming more educated and, relieved from the obligations of multiple childbearing, were beginning to agitate for universal suffrage. Some were applying to medical school, which Storer adamantly opposed.[24]

The medical profession, by adopting and promoting a more scientific approach to disease, was now burnished with a better public image. With its rising stature, it became increasingly influential in legislatures, so that a steadily increasing number of states passed antiabortion laws, varying in detail but ultimately making abortion a criminal offense from the time of conception. By 1900, every state had an antiabortion law and the eclipse was complete.

It is ironic that the medical profession was the prime mover in the antiabortion movement, for paradoxically, it is estimated that today more than 60% of physicians favor a liberal attitude toward termination of pregnancy.

Roe v. Wade

The earth-shaking 1973 decision of the United States Supreme Court dramatically changed the landscape of abortion. A carnival sideshow barker, Norma L. McCorvey, finding herself pregnant, chose to allege that she had been raped to take advantage of a legal exception in Texas antiabortion law. Her plea, declined for lack of evidence, rendered her unable to terminate her pregnancy, so she sought the legal advice of attorneys Linda Coffee and Sarah Weddington who, in turn, filed on her behalf suit in U.S. District Court in Texas under

---

24   "I am no advocate of unwomanly woman. I would not transplant them from their God-given sphere, to the pulpit, the forum, or the cares of state nor would I repeat the experiment…of females attempting the practice of the medical profession."

the alias of Jane Roe. The defendant in the suit was Dallas County District Court Attorney Henry Wade. The court found in favor of McCorvey, the merits of the case based on the IX Amendment, or Bill of Rights, and the 1965 decision in Griswold v. Connecticut on the right to privacy, but justices declined to grant an injunction against enforcement of current Texas law. As is well known, the case was reviewed by the U.S. Supreme Court, and on 22nd January, 1973, by a 7 to 2 majority, supported the opinion written by Justice Harry Blackmun, who based his arguments not on the IX amendment, but on the XIV amendment guaranteeing the right to privacy based on the Due Process Clause.

The defining section of the decision was Section X, stating that during the first trimester, the state cannot restrict a woman's right to abortion; in the second trimester the state may only regulate the abortion procedure "in ways that are reasonably related to maternal health." During the third trimester, the state can choose to restrict or proscribe abortion as it sees fit when the fetus is viable ("except when necessary, in appropriate medical judgment, for the preservation of the life or health of the mother").

Statistics in abortion in the United States show that in 2005 there were 1.21 million abortions performed in the nation out of some 6.4 million pregnancies. This amounts to approximately 19 abortions per 1,000 women, a decline from a peak of 29/1,000 in 1981. Typically most (90%) take place during the first trimester in women who are, for the most part, under 25 years old (50.4%) and are unmarried (86%). Many are poor, with 27% living under the poverty line.

With 90% of abortions taking place in the first 12 weeks of conception, unless one equates a 12-centimeter fetus with a live birth, the accusation of infanticide used as an argument against abortion is invalid. Since most women seeking abortion are single and poor, it makes little sense from a social or economic point of view to insist on carriage to term. Women who are poor and single make poor candidates for parenthood. No doubt the controversy over abortion will persist, but armed with facts, there seems little to sustain the position of antiabortionists.

Bibliography

Chapter One: The Reformer – Anthony Comstock

_____ The Comstock Law. Forty-second Congress. Sess. III. CH.258. 1873.

_____ "Message from the Senate, notifying the House of passage of S. No.1572 for suppression of trade in circulation of obscene literature and articles of immoral use, etc." Congressional Globe. 22 Feb. 1873, p.1638

Beisel, Nicola Kay. Imperiled Innocents: Anthony Comstock and Family Reproduction in Victorian America. Princeton, NJ: Princeton UP, 1997.

Bennett, De Robigne Mortimer, De Robigne Mortimer Bennett, and De Robigne Mortimer Bennett. Anthony Comstock: His Career of Cruelty and Crime. New York: Da Capo, 1971.

Bradford, Roderick. "The Truth Seeker D.M. Bennett: the 19th century's most controversial publisher and American Free Speech Martyr." American Atheist Magazine. Winter, 2004.

Bradford, Roderick. "The Truth Seeker on Trial: United States vs D. M. Bennett, Mar. 20, 1879." Retrieved from Hackwriters.com.

Broun, Heywood, and Margaret Leech. Anthony Comstock, Roundsman of the Lord. New York: A. & C. Boni, 1927.

Hopkins, Mary Alden. "Birth Control and Public Morals: An interview with Anthony Comstock." Harper's Weekly. 22 May 1915: pp. 489-90.

Horowitz, Helen Lefkowitz. "Victoria Woodhull, Anthony Comstock, and Conflict over Sex in the United States in the 1870s." The Journal of American History Vol. 87, No. 2 (Sep., 2000): pp. 403-434.

Mandelbaum, Seymour J. "Mme Restell." Notable American Women. Cambridge: Belknap Press, 1971.

Meriam, C. L. "Speech of Hon. C.L. Meriam in support of S. No. 1572." Appendix to Congressional Globe. 1 Mar. 1873: p.168.

Trumbull, Charles G. Anthony Comstock, Fighter; Some Impressions of a Lifetime Adventure in Conflict with the Powers of Evil. New York: Fleming H. Revell, 1913.

Chapter Two: The Nurse
Margaret Louise (Higgins) Sanger

Chesler, Ellen. Woman of Valor: Margaret Sanger and the Birth Control Movement in America. New York, London, Toronto and Sydney: Simon and Schuster,1992

Gray, Madeline. Margaret Sanger; a Biography. New York: Richard Marek,1979.

Katz,Esther, ed. Selected Papers of Margaret Sanger. Vol.1: The Woman Rebel. Urbana and Chicago: University of Illinois Press, 2003.

Kennedy, David M. Birth Control in America; The Career of Margaret Sanger. New Haven and London: Yale University Press, 1970.

Rose, June. Marie Stopes and the Sexual Revolution. London: Faber and Faber, 1992.

Sanger, Margaret. My Fight for Birth Control. New York: Farrar and Rinehart, 1931.

Sanger, Margaret. The Autobiography. Mineola, New York: Dover Publications, 1971.

Chapter Three: Physiology

Kistner, Robert William. Gynecology: Principles and Practice, Hormonal Aspect of Menstruation. Chicago: Year Book Medical Publishers, 1971.

Parsons, Langdon and Sommers, Sheldon C. Gynecology: The Menstrual Cycle. Philadelphia: Saunders,1969.

Chapter Four: The Biologists
Dr. Gregory Pincus and Dr. Min Chueh Chang

Bennett, John P. Chemical Contraception. New York and London: Columbia University Press, 1974.

Chang, M.C. and Pincus, G. "The effects of progesterone and related compounds on ovulation and early development in the rabbit." Acta physiol. Latinoam. 3 (1953):177.

Chang, M.C., Pincus, G. and Rock, John. "Effects of certain 19-nor steroids on reproductive processes and fertility." Federation Proceedings Dec.1959: p. 18.

Garcia, Celson Ramon, Pincus, G. and Rock, John. "Synthetic progestins in the normal human menstrual cycle: Recent progress in hormone research." New York: Presented at the Laurentian Conference: Academic Vol X111 (1956).

Garcia, Celson Ramon, Pincus, G., and Rock, John. "Effects of certain 19-nor steroids on the normal human menstrual cycle." Science 124 (1956): 891.

Garcia, Celson Ramon, Pincus, G. and Rock, John. "Effects of 3 19-nor steroids on human ovulation and menstruation." American Journal of Obstetrics and Gynecology 75 (Jan. 1958): 82.

Makepeace, A.W. "Weinstein and Friedman: The Effect of Progestin and Progesterone on Ovulation in the Rabbit." American Journal of Physiology. 1937.

Pincus, G. "Some effects of Progesterone and Related Compounds upon Reproduction and early Development in Mammals." Acta Enocrinologica Vol 28 (1956).

Slechta, Robert F. M.S. "Chang M.C.Ph.D. & Pincus G. Sc.D.: Effects of Progesterone and Related Compounds on Mating and Pregnancy in the Rat." Fertility and Sterility. Vol 5 (1954): 282-293.

Speroff, Leonard. A Good Man: Gregory Goodwin Pincus: The man, his story, the birth control pill. Portland, Oregon: Arnica Publishing, 2009.

Chapter Five: The Chemists – Russell Marker, Carl Djerassi, George Rosenkranz, Luis Miramontes and Frank Colton

Absell, Bernard. The Pill: A biography of the drug that changed the world. Two interviews with Russell Marker (State College, PA, spring and summer 1991). New York City: Random House, 1995.

Djerassi, Carl. This Man's Pill: Reflections on the fiftieth birthday of the pill. Interview with Russell Marker (3 Oct. 1979). Oxford: Oxford University Press, 2003.

Lehmann, P.,Bolivar, A.; Quintero, R., "Russell Marker, Pioneer of the Mexican Steroid Industry." Journal of Chemical Education 50:3 (March 1973).

Marker, Russell. Autobiographical Notes. Pennsylvania State University: Pattee Library, 1969.

Marker, Russell. Transcript of Interview conducted by Jeffrey Sturchio at Pennsylvania State University on 17th April 1987. Philadelphia: Chemical Heritage Foundation(Oral History Program), 2001.

Yarmey, Kristen. Labors and Legacies: the Chemists of Penn State. Philadelphia: Pennsylvania State University, 2006.

Chapter Six: The Financier Katharine Dexter McCormick

Fields, Armond. Katharine Dexter McCormick: Pioneer for women's rights. Santa Barbara: Praeger Publishing House, 2003.

Chapter Seven: The Journalist
Dr. Ernest Gruening ....

Gruening, Ernest. Many Battles. New York City: Liveright, 1973.

Chapter Eight: The Puerto Rican Field Studies ....

De Areallano, A.B. Ramirez and Seipp, Conrad. Colonialism, Catholicism and Contraception: A History of Birth Control in Puerto Rico." Chapel Hill: University of North Carolina Press, 1983.

Chapter Nine: The Gynecologist
Dr. John Rock ....

_____ Proceedings of a Symposium on 19-Nor Progestational Steroids. Searle Research Laboratories, 1957.

Garcia, Celson Ramon; Rock, John; and Pincus, Gregory. "Synthetic Progestins in the Normal Human Menstrual Cycle." Recent Progress in Hormone Research. Laurentian Conference (presented 1956).

Garcia, Celson Ramon; Rock, John; and Pincus, Gregory. "Effects of Certain 19-Nor Steroids on the Normal Human Menstrual Cycle." Science, 2 Nov. 1956.

Garcia, Celson Ramon; Rock, John; and Pincus, Gregory. "Effects of Certain Nor-Steroids on Reproductive Processes and Fertility." Laurentian Conference (presented 1957).

Garcia, Celson Ramon; Rock, John; and Pincus, Gregory. "Effects of Three 19-Nor Steroids on Human Ovulation and Menstruation." American Journal of Obstetrics and Gynecology, January 1958.

Marsh, Margaret S. and Ronner, Wanda. The Fertility Doctor. Baltimore: Johns Hopkins University Press, 2008.

McLaughlin, Loretta. The Pill, John Rock and the Church. New York City: Little, Brown and co., 1982.

Pincus, Gregory. The Control of Fertility. Maryland Heights: Academic Press,1965.

Pincus, Gregory; Rock, John; Celson Ramon Garcia; Edris Rice Wray MD; Manuel Paniagua MD; with Iris Rodriguez B.S. "Fertility Control with Oral Medication." American Journal of Obstetrics and Gynecology, June 1958.

Rock, John. The Time Has Come: A Catholic doctor's proposals to end the battle over birth control. New York City: Alfred Knopf, 1964.

Chapter Ten: Epilogue

Vessey MP, Doll R. "Investigation of relation between use of oral contraceptives and thromboembolic disease." BMJ 2 (1968): 199-205.

Centers for Disease Control. Oral contraceptives and Cancer Risk. MMWR, 30.July 1982.

U.S. Supreme Court 381 U.S. 479 (Griswold v. Connecticut).

_____ Birth rates, fertility rates and population growth: U.S. statistics.

World Population Graph. United Nations Environmental Program.

President's Emergency Plan for AIDS Relief. United States Government. http://www.pepfar.gov. 21 Aug. 2011.

Riddle, John. Contraception and Abortion from the Ancient World to the Renaissance. Cambridge: Harvard University Press, 1994.

Mohr, James. Abortion in America. Oxford: Oxford University Press, 1978.

Supreme Court of the United States: 401 U.S. 113 (Roe v. Wade).

"A Sad Day for Science at the FDA." New England Journal of Medicine, 2005; 353:2619-2621

National Vital Statistics System. U.S. Department of Health and Human Services, Centers for Disease Control and Prevention National Center for Health Statistics.

Marchbanks, et al. "Oral contraceptives and the risk of breast cancer." New England Journal of Medicine, 2002; 346:2025-2032.

"Abortion." Guttmacher Institute. http://www.guttmacher.org/ sections/abortion.php. Retrieved 21 Aug. 2011.

Index

Symbols

A

B

E

F

G

H

I

International Harvester, 96, 104

International Malthusian and Birth Control Organization, 45

Isabella of Spain, 9

J

Jacobs, Dr. Aletta, 30, 45, 157

Jacobs, Dr. Walter, 71

Japanese Medical Association, 210

Johns Hopkins, 47, 190, 235

Jones Act, 141, 154

Journal of the American Chemical Society, 68, 89

K

Kaiser Wilhelm Institute, 58

Keller, Helen, 114

Kendall, Edward, 91

Kennedy, Anne, 124, 128

Kennedy, Joseph, 192

Kennedy, Rose, 192

Kenyon College, 88

Kharasch, Morris, 67, 68

Knox, John, 9

L

Laboratorios Hormonos, 79, 80

La Democracia, 155

LaGuardia, Fiorello, 136

Lally, Monsignor Francis, 193

Lambeth Conference, 46

La Prensa, 119, 120, 121

M

N

Parres, José, 127

Patrick Steptoe, Bravister and Edwards, 57

Pennsylvania State University, 69, 234

Pennsylvania, University of, 200

Pfizer, 64, 182

Pierson, Dr. Richard, 102

Pincus, Dr. Gregory, 8, 55, 56, 57, 58, 59, 60, 63, 64, 92, 104, 105, 106, 107, 109, 148, 171, 172, 174, 175, 177, 179, 180, 181, 182, 183, 196, 197, 201, 202, 207, 233, 234, 235, 236

Pius XI, Pope, 46, 193

Planned Parenthood Federation of America, 103

Pomona College, 181

Pond building, 75

Pons, Dr. Juan, 176, 177

Portet, Lorenzo, 31, 32, 39

Portland Evening News, 131, 133, 135, 136

Portland, ME, 34, 130, 131, 133, 135, 136, 234

pregneneolone, 74

Press Herald, 130

progesterone, 53, 54, 55, 60, 61, 62, 63, 65, 71, 72, 73, 74, 75, 78, 79, 80, 81, 82, 83, 84, 86, 87, 89, 90, 92, 105, 106, 107, 171, 174, 194, 195, 196, 197, 198, 204, 233

Psychology of Sex, 29

Puerto, Felipe Carillo, 128

Puerto Rican Emergency Relief Fund (PRERA), 161, 163, 164, 165

Puerto Rican Medical Association, 164

Puerto Rican Reconstruction Administration (PRRA), 142, 146, 148, 165, 167

Puerto Rico, University of, 143, 144, 160, 171, 200

pulmonary embolus, 211

Purity Congress, 19

Q

R

V

W

Y

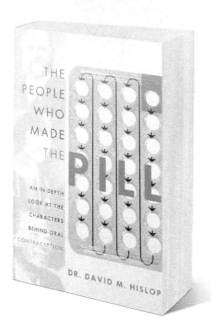

How can you use this book?

MOTIVATE

EDUCATE

THANK

INSPIRE

PROMOTE

CONNECT

Why have a custom version of *The People Who Made the Pill?*

- Build personal bonds with customers, prospects, employees, donors, and key constituencies

- Develop a long-lasting reminder of your event, milestone, or celebration

- Provide a keepsake that inspires change in behavior and change in lives

- Deliver the ultimate "thank you" gift that remains on coffee tables and bookshelves

- Generate the "wow" factor

Books are thoughtful gifts that provide a genuine sentiment that other promotional items cannot express. They promote employee discussions and interaction, reinforce an event's meaning or location, and they make a lasting impression. Use your book to say "Thank You" and show people that you care.